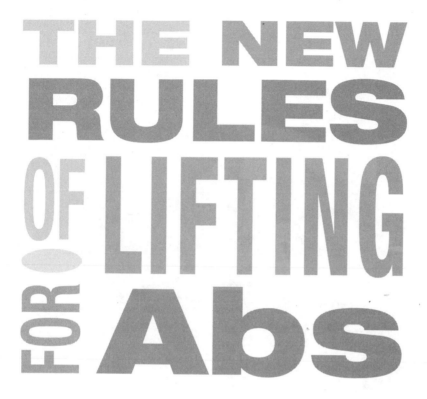

THE NEW RULES OF LIFTING FOR Abs

THE NEW RULES OF LIFTING FOR Abs

A Myth-Busting Fitness Plan for Men and Women Who Want a Strong Core and a Pain-Free Back

Lou Schuler and **Alwyn Cosgrove**

AVERY
A MEMBER OF PENGUIN GROUP (USA) INC.
NEW YORK

Published by the Penguin Group
Penguin Group (USA) Inc., 375 Hudson Street, New York, New York 10014, USA ·
Penguin Group (Canada), 90 Eglinton Avenue East, Suite 700, Toronto, Ontario M4P 2Y3, Canada
(a division of Pearson Penguin Canada Inc.) · Penguin Books Ltd, 80 Strand, London WC2R 0RL, England ·
Penguin Ireland, 25 St Stephen's Green, Dublin 2, Ireland (a division of Penguin Books Ltd) ·
Penguin Group (Australia), 250 Camberwell Road, Camberwell, Victoria 3124, Australia
(a division of Pearson Australia Group Pty Ltd) · Penguin Books India Pvt Ltd, 11 Community Centre,
Panchsheel Park, New Delhi–110 017, India · Penguin Group (NZ), 67 Apollo Drive, Rosedale,
North Shore 0632, New Zealand (a division of Pearson New Zealand Ltd) ·
Penguin Books (South Africa) (Pty) Ltd, 24 Sturdee Avenue, Rosebank, Johannesburg 2196, South Africa

Penguin Books Ltd, Registered Offices: 80 Strand, London WC2R 0RL, England

First trade paperback edition 2012

Illustrations on pages 16 and 17 are by Ines Fripp; they are taken from *Human Anatomy for Art Students* (1911).

Most Avery books are available at special quantity discounts for bulk purchase for sales promotions, premiums, fund-
raising, and educational needs. Special books or book excerpts also can be created to fit specific needs. For details, write
Penguin Group (USA) Inc. Special Markets, 375 Hudson Street, New York, NY 10014.

The Library of Congress catalogued the hardcover edition as follows:

Schuler, Lou.
The new rules of lifting for abs : a myth-busting fitness plan for men and women who
want a strong core and a pain-free back / Lou Schuler and Alwyn Cosgrove.
p.   cm.
ISBN 978-1-58333-413-3
1. Weight lifting.   2. Abdominal exercises.   3. Muscle strength.   I. Cosgrove, Alwyn.   II. Title.
GV546.3.S38   2010   2010029290
796.41—dc22

ISBN 978-1-58333-460-7 (paperback edition)

Printed in the United States of America
1   3   5   7   9   10   8   6   4   2

BOOK DESIGN BY TANYA MAIBORODA

Acknowledgments

EVERY BOOK I write is a synthesis of ideas from more coaches, scientists, and enthusiasts than I could ever remember, much less acknowledge. So I'll start by expressing my gratitude to my coauthor, Alwyn Cosgrove, for his relentless pursuit of the best training methods, and for his willingness to translate those methods to this format so our readers can benefit. The workouts in *The New Rules of Lifting for Abs* aren't exactly what you'd get if you were being coached by Alwyn or the trainers at Results Fitness, but they're the next best thing.

Second, I want to thank the readers of *The New Rules of Lifting* and *The New Rules of Lifting for Women*. I've corresponded with thousands of you over the years, and the questions you ask and concerns you express are always the jumping-off point for each book I write.

I'm lucky to work with the best colleagues a fitness author could possibly have: my editor, Megan Newman, along with Miriam Rich, and the rest of the team at Avery; my agent, David Black; publicist Gregg Stebben; and photographer Michael Tedesco, who deserves a special thanks for his role in this project. This is the most ambitious book we've done in the *NROL* series so far, in terms of the number of exercises and the complexity involved in shooting them. Michael pulled together a true all-star team for the project, including assistants Michael Lorenzini and Danelle Manthey and models Kim Strother and Joe Kavitski. Many thanks also go to the management and trainers at Velocity Sports Performance and the Human Performance Center in Allentown, Pennsylvania: Jeff Hewlings, Mike Cerimele, Chris Leavy, and Brian Zarbatany, along with all the coaches, athletes, and clients who tolerated our disruptive presence with patience and good humor.

Thanks also to Rob Milani at Perform Better for providing some of the equipment you see in the photos, and to Karen Hatzigeorgiou (karenswhimsy.com) for the scans of the anatomical illustrations in Chapter 2.

Finally, I want to thank Kimberly, my wife, who took on the role of caterer for the two-day shoot, in addition to the full-time job of wrangling our three children and running our household.

This book is dedicated to Harrison, our firstborn, who had visible abs the day he arrived, and still has them now.

—L.S.

A SPECIAL THANKS has to go to Lou Schuler. About twelve years ago he met a young Scottish immigrant in New York who was working as a personal trainer, and he saw something that maybe no one else saw. Thank you for believing in me, and for all the opportunities that have since come my way because of you.

To Adam Campbell: I'll be forever grateful for the opportunities you gave me to communicate my ideas to more people than I ever could have reached on my own.

To all the lecturers, coaches, authors, and seminar hosts I've learned from over the years: My growth has come, in part, from your willingness to teach. I'll continue to pay it forward.

To the Perform Better team, who gave me an opportunity to share what we do at Results Fitness with a wider audience: Thank you.

To Derek Campbell, my original mentor: You changed the direction of my life. I want to be just like you when I grow up!

To my family at Results Fitness: None of this is possible without you guys. I am by far the worst trainer at my own facility, and I'm very proud of that.

To my mum: I hope you're watching. To my dad and Derek, my brother: Thanks for being the base from which I launched.

To God, and in no small part the elite team of doctors and nurses at UCLA Medical Center who saved my life and gave me these extra days here: I don't know why I deserve these days, but I will never waste them and will always treat them as a gift. If it weren't for you, this book wouldn't have my name on it.

And as always to my soul mate, Rachel: You're the most amazing thing that's ever happened to me. Thanks for everything.

—A.C.

Contents

Introduction:
If a Tree Falls on
My Shoulder . . .

MY PROBLEMS STARTED with a tree. It was December 2006, about a month before my fiftieth birthday. The tree had fallen over into a neighbor's yard, and like a good neighbor, I broke out my little chain saw and went to work cutting the tree into pieces small enough to carry to my woodpile a couple hundred feet away.

I was in terrific shape at the time. In the gym, I regularly trained with weights that were close to my all-time bests. Outside the gym, I felt strong enough to tackle anything a suburban family guy would ever be called upon to do.

Like, say, a fallen tree.

My plucky little chain saw quit on me before I finished sawing the tree down to size. That left me with a chunk of trunk that, I'd estimate, was at least a hundred pounds—certainly not beyond my strength, but awkward as hell to manage. I stood it upright, leaned it against my shoulder, lifted it off the ground, and started toward the woodpile.

I made it halfway across the lawn before it slipped and landed on my picnic table. The fact that it smashed the picnic table like dry kindling should've been a hint that perhaps I needed to revisit the strategy of carrying it the rest of the way.

Alas, I ignored both my body and the evidence of the crushed table, and instead picked it up again. This time I carried the log over my right shoulder, which, like the picnic table, has never been the same. I didn't break, tear, or dislocate anything that I know of. I didn't need surgery. I simply lost strength and my pain-free range of motion, despite hundreds of sets of corrective exercises and the best efforts of a talented physical therapist.

A year later, a small hernia emerged on the right side of my lower abdomen. There was no need for surgery, but, as with the shoulder problem, my strength declined almost immediately.

A few months after that, I hurt my right knee doing one-legged squats in the gym. I limped around for six months before I finally sought the help of a soft-tissue specialist, who dug his thumbs into my leg muscles until he flattened out the knots and restored my range of motion. The reprieve lasted a week or two before I tore a muscle in my right calf while coaching my daughter's soccer team.

So there I was, in the fall of 2008, wondering what I'd done to produce this chain of injuries on the right side of my body. I'd been working out since I was thirteen. Everything about me—my career, my hobbies, my friendships, my wardrobe, the way I carried myself, even my parenting style—was based at least in part on my lifelong enthusiasm for physical activity in general, and strength training in particular. And now my body was telling me to try something else.

If you've read either or both of the previous books in the New Rules of Lifting series, you know how I structured my workouts: minimal warm-up, followed by forty-five minutes to an hour in the weight room. I included a lot of variety in my programs—when you have the privilege of working with Alwyn Cosgrove, as creative a coauthor as any fitness-book writer could hope to find, there's always something new to try. But the structure hadn't changed in years.

My new workouts were radically different. I started with a dynamic warm-up routine that developed and then maintained mobility, flexibility, and balanced strength in my lower body. I found myself doing exercises for muscles I'd never actively trained in nearly forty years of lifting. The routines were complex, but the goal was simple: I didn't ever again want to develop muscle knots that required the intervention of a therapist's thumbs.

The next part of the workout was devoted to core exercises. Without any particular plan, I did everything I thought would help me compensate for the torn curtain in my abdominal wall. When exercises started to feel too easy, I either found a way to make them more challenging, or I moved on to something new. I discovered that when I did these mid-body exercises near the beginning of my workouts, instead of at the end, I was able to do them with more intensity and better attention to form, and consequently got more out of them than I ever had before.

Only then—typically fifteen to twenty minutes into my workout—did I cross over to the weight room. I was extremely limited in what I could do at first. My shoulder injury made bench presses an exercise in masochism; even push-ups hurt. Heavy squats were out of the question, thanks to my aching and fragile knees, and the hernia gave me a healthy fear of maximum-load deadlifts.

These weight routines rarely went longer than twenty minutes, which meant my total gym time was thirty-five to forty minutes. I did this three days a week.

Logic says I should've gotten disappointing results. With the loss of strength, the narrow range of exercise choices, the extended warm-up routine, and the reduced time in the weight room, I should've gotten weaker, smaller, and fatter.

But I didn't. My strength stabilized. I replaced some of the muscle I lost. And most amazing of all, I got *leaner*. Clothes fit better. People who hadn't seen me in a while commented on my slimmer physique.

I tried to figure out what could account for this unexpected result. Was I eating less? Perhaps. (I'll explore ways to time meals and avoid overeating in Part 4.) Was I under less stress? No. If anything, I had more than usual during that time. Was I exercising more outside the gym? Yes. Besides coaching soccer, I played baseball on a team for the first time since I was twelve. (I'll talk about outside-the-gym activity throughout the book.)

The simplest explanation is probably best. If you eat a little less food and get a little more physical activity, of course you'll end up with a little less fat.

That, however, led to another, more important question: *Why* was I getting more exercise? I had started near zero; in the summer and fall of 2008, I had trouble walking, and running was out of the question. But by the summer of 2009, I was lighter and faster than I'd been in years, if not decades. Seriously: In my final baseball game of the season, I actually beat out an infield single, something I couldn't do when I was twelve. (Then again, when I was twelve I *occasionally* hit the ball out of the infield. So there's that.)

The fact that I was moving more, and moving better, seemed directly related to the fact that I *could* move more, and *could* move better. Clearly, I thought, that's a benefit of this new workout system. It restored functional abilities, making me faster and more athletic.

But I still wondered if there was something about these workouts that allowed me to burn more calories in the gym, even though I was spending less time in the weight room, and using lighter weights when I was there. The workouts weren't easy; I was constantly pushing the limits of my balance, coordination, and core strength. Maybe, I thought, I'm using more muscles, or using the same ones differently.

MORE THAN A HUNCH

Meanwhile, three thousand miles away, Alwyn was changing the way he trained his clients at Results Fitness, the gym he owns with his wife, Rachel, in Santa Clarita, California. Alwyn realized his clients were coming to him in worse shape than they had just a few years before. Many didn't get enough movement outside the gym to cover even the bare minimum of their conditioning needs. The hours they spent hunched over laptops and iPhones distorted their posture. And the lack of physical activity, combined with the need to spend ever-longer hours working on ever-smaller communication devices, meant they required remedial work on mobility and core strength.

Even the clients who came to Alwyn "in shape"—they'd been exercising regularly and weren't overweight—tended to have unbalanced fitness. They might have great mobility from yoga, or terrific endurance from running or cycling, but surprisingly little strength. Others were strong, but with dangerously deficient core endurance and stability. And some had gotten the memo about core training, but had developed it at the expense of strength, power, mobility, and overall conditioning.

So Alwyn developed a new workout configuration to better serve his clients, one that was similar to the program I'd pieced together to accommodate and rehabilitate my string of injuries. Of course it was much more sophisticated than mine—that's why he's the coach and I'm the writer—but the goals and principles were the same.

None of this would be worth describing at length if it weren't for one crucial detail: *The new workouts are more effective than the way we used to do things.* Alwyn's clients get leaner and more athletic, they look better and feel better, and they achieve those results faster than they did before.

That's why we decided it was time to write *The New Rules of Lifting for Abs.*

THE A LIST

You may wonder why it took this long for me to use the A word. I've mentioned core training. I've talked about getting leaner and improving overall conditioning. But I haven't yet told you why "abs" appears in the title of the book.

Good question.

"Abs" is an evocative word. If we stop to think about it, we know it describes the muscles that reside on the front of your torso between your ribs and pelvis. But when we don't stop to think, it means a lot more than that. In just three letters, it describes a muscular ideal, a blend of physical power combined with disciplined conditioning. A person with visible abs, male or female, is assumed to be strong, fast, athletic, and durable. Just as we're shocked to see accomplished athletes with flab hanging over their waistlines, we don't expect someone with a well-defined midsection to bail out halfway through a job, a game, or a training session.

We assume they're good; if they weren't, they wouldn't have abs.

That's a lot of meaning for such a little word.

To pay off on our title, Alwyn and I know we need to deliver more than the standard bunches-of-crunches approach to ab training. Building those muscles is important, no question, but it's useless in isolation. That's why *NROL for Abs* offers a full-spectrum conditioning system designed to help you become stronger, leaner, more muscular, and more athletic.

You'll do it with four-part workouts:

Dynamic warm-ups help you awaken and activate your muscles, while ensuring that your most vulnerable joints have their optimal range of motion.

Core training builds balanced stability, endurance, and strength in your abs, lower back, and hips.

Strength training—aka weight lifting—increases your strength (obviously), power, and muscle mass.

Metabolic work burns fat and improves your overall conditioning.

Although each of the four components focuses on a separate and crucial aspect of fitness, the success of the system depends on their common benefits. All of them help make you stronger, leaner, more muscular, more athletic, and better conditioned. All of them help you look, move, and feel better. And all of them contribute to a smaller, flatter, and more aesthetically appealing waistline.

Perhaps most important, all of them help you reverse the ravages of modern life—the long commutes, the crushing deadlines, the horrors of the modern food supply.

ABOHOLICS ANONYMOUS

All that said, I understand that a lot of you reading this picked up *NROL for Abs* because you're looking for a collection of ab-training exercises. You've come to the right place. Alwyn has provided dozens of them, divided into three categories, which I'll explain in Chapter 3. Whether you're a beginner or a lifelong gym rat, I'm confident you'll find exercises you haven't tried before. Many include progressions from the easiest to the most challenging variations.

If you came to this book looking for Alwyn's latest workout programs, again, you won't be disappointed. Along with the core exercises, you'll find a total-body training system that you can use for the next three to six months, and then repeat as many times as you want. Each time you do the three-stage program, you can choose more advanced versions of many of the exercises, making every workout a fresh and unique challenge.

In fact, I'll go out on a limb and say this: Just about anybody who's serious about training, or wants to be, will find something in *NROL for Abs* that's new and intriguing.

The dedicated lifter: If you're a guy who's been working out vigorously and consistently for years, chances are good that, like me, you developed strength and size at the expense of other important, functional qualities. Or maybe, like me, you woke up one day to realize that your body could no longer do some of the things that made you bigger and stronger than the average guy. You need a program that offers full-spectrum fitness.

The cardio queen: For you, the perfect workout is a couple of laps around the circuit of machines in your gym, followed by an hour on the treadmill. You lost a few pounds when you started that program eleven years ago, but since then you've gained weight in all the wrong places, despite trying every diet plan to hit the *New York Times* bestseller list. Meanwhile, you've avoided serious strength training because you feared getting "too big." Now you're ready to concede that no matter how many hours you spend on that treadmill, you've already gotten all the benefits it offers. It's time for something new.

The perpetual beginner: Every health club in America is populated by men and women who start a new training program on January 2 (our National Day of Retonement), but give up by March 17 (the official end of "fitness season"). You can tell you're one of these people if you reveal to friends and family members the exact date on which you plan to start your next program.

Each year, you encounter the same problem: The program you choose offers limited benefits, and once you've achieved them, you quickly lose interest. You need a training program you can stick to for months rather than weeks, one that delivers the kind of results that keep you motivated.

The chunky monkey: I had abs before they were cool. Every now and then I'll see a picture of myself from my late teens or early twenties, and I'm almost as surprised by the six-pack abs as I am by the full head of hair. I did sit-ups and crunches, of course, along with push-ups and pull-ups and anything else I could do without a gym membership. But what I really wanted was to be bigger. I achieved that goal in my middle to late thirties, but at the expense of my waistline. Some of the pictures from back then are as surprising as the ones from my days of follicular abundance, but in a bad way. Even my face looks fat.

So if you're devoted to exercise, but don't actually look like you work out, I can relate. You may get more out of *NROL for Abs* than any other category of reader, in terms of visible results. You have a base of training experience and knowledge, along with some hard-earned muscle beneath all that collateral fat, which will help you push yourself through Alwyn's workouts to achieve the maximum benefits.

The specialist: Maybe you're a marathoner or triathlete. Maybe you're a yoga enthusiast. Maybe you're a martial artist, or a weekend soccer player or golfer, or a Civil War reenactor whose army gets stuck marching uphill more often than not. You have a strong base of endurance or flexibility or athleticism or commitment to historical accuracy (there weren't many fat guys in either army in the 1860s) and unwavering dedication to your sport or activity.

You need a workout system that complements your chosen sport, without forcing you to choose one over the other. You know you'll be a better soccer or basketball or tennis player if you're lighter, leaner, and stronger. You know you'll have less risk of injury if you improve the mobility of the joints that need it and the stability of the joints that don't. (You'll learn more about this in Chapter 9.) And no matter how much you enjoy your sport, you know it creates muscle and strength imbalances that, left uncorrected, will set you up for serious problems down the road, if they haven't already.

THE STANDARD DISCLAIMERS

So who might be disappointed? Alwyn's workout system isn't designed for serious bodybuilders or powerlifters, or for high-level competitive athletes. It isn't meant for people whose primary goal is to put on extreme amounts of muscle, or to increase strength and sport-specific performance in a dramatic, boundary-pushing way. Alwyn has on many occasions trained clients to reach those goals, using elements of this system. But if you're looking to push yourself to the outer limits of your genetic potential, you'll need a program and diet specific to that goal.

I should also note here that *NROL for Abs* isn't a "weight loss" book. It belongs in the "body composition" category—books with workout and nutrition information designed to help you improve your body's ratio of fat to muscle. You can accomplish this by building muscle without adding fat, shedding fat without losing muscle, or achieving the Holy Grail of muscle growth combined with fat loss.

The main focus is on fat loss through intense exercise (make no mistake: Alwyn's workouts are tough), lifestyle changes, and diet modification. There's no formal *NROL* diet; I've written books with and without complete meal plans, and readers seem to achieve similar results on both. The last one had a complete diet plan, and the next one may as well. This one doesn't. Instead, it offers tips and strategies based on the latest research and the most successful techniques used by professionals and enthusiasts.

But I know before the book is even published that I'll hear from readers who either gained a lot of muscle or lost an unfathomable amount of weight. You might be one of them. People who are willing to try something new and dedicate themselves to it for months or years often achieve extraordinary results. Readers using Alwyn's *NROL* programs have told me about results that far surpass anything I've ever achieved on any program I've tried in a lifetime of lifting. If I weren't so happy for them I might get jealous.

So what results will you achieve with *NROL for Abs*? I look forward to hearing about them. Until then, I hope you enjoy the benefits of our new approach to training. It took a fallen tree to steer me in this direction. I'll be very happy if you can get all the benefits of what I learned without anything falling on you.

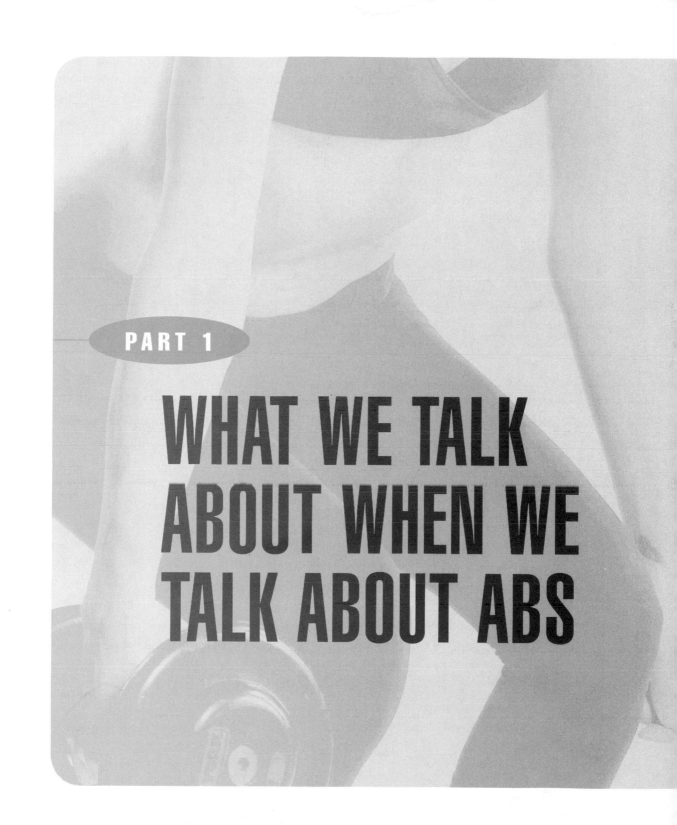

PART 1

WHAT WE TALK ABOUT WHEN WE TALK ABOUT ABS

So Where Are Those Abs You've Been Promised?

YOUR GYM, SIX P.M. MONDAY. You find an unoccupied strip of carpet in the area reserved for warming up and doing ab exercises.

The guy to your right is on his back with his feet in the air, spasmodically cranking out crunch after crunch, jerking his knees toward his chin and his chin toward his knees on every repetition.

The woman to your left is doing a plank exercise, with her weight resting on her forearms and toes. But she doesn't seem to understand that a plank is supposed to be flat. The area between her shoulders and butt more realistically resembles a trench.

The ambitious young man across the room does shoulder presses with five-pound dumbbells while balancing on a Bosu ball, a plastic platform mounted on half of an inflated sphere.

And then there's the hard-core bodybuilder guy on the other side of the gym. He's doing full-range-of-motion sit-ups on a slant board while holding a twenty-five-pound weight plate against his chest.

If you took a survey, the bodybuilder would tell you he's working his "abs." Bowing

Bridget and Bosu Bill would tell you they're training the "core." And with Crunching Carl, there's an even chance of getting either answer.

Of the four, the bodybuilder has given the best answer. He is indeed working his major abdominal muscles, although he's doing it in one of the most dangerous ways possible.

The others? Bridget certainly has the right idea; the plank is one of the best entry-level exercises for working the cylinder of mid-body muscles that comprise your body's core. The problem is that she's undercutting her effort with terrible form.

Bill, on the other hand, is doing an exercise that would only be effective for him if he's rehabilitating an injury. Otherwise, he'd be much better off doing his shoulder presses with his feet on the ground and much heavier dumbbells in his hands. Not only would that provide a better challenge to his core muscles; assuming he does the exercise with good posture, it would build far more strength and muscle mass in his shoulders and arms.

And Carl? Let's just say he really, really needs to know these new rules.

NEW RULE #1 • The most important role of the abdominal muscles is to protect your spine.

You know those childhood nightmares you had every year around Halloween, the ones where you were attacked by homicidal skeletons? Totally couldn't happen. Take away the dozens of muscles that support the spine and that once-scary skeleton would collapse under the weight of its own calcified remains. The mere act of walking generates seven times the amount of compressive force needed to buckle the spine. A spinal column without its supporting structures—all those muscles and connective tissues that attach to it—is truly a bridge to nowhere.

And yet the human body is capable of amazing feats of strength and athleticism. We lift heavy objects off the ground. We play sports that require us to run, jump, throw, catch, change directions, and occasionally get knocked to the ground by an opponent. We do these things without stopping to think about whether or not our spinal column can support the load, absorb the impact, or survive the challenge. That's because our muscles and connective tissues, when healthy and well trained, do an extraordinary job of keeping our spine in a safe and stable position.

NEW RULE #2 • You can't protect your spine by doing exercises that damage it.

Our ideas about training abdominal muscles are heavily influenced by Stuart McGill, Ph.D., a professor of spine mechanics at the University of Waterloo, in Ontario, and probably the most often cited expert on exercise and back injury. I quoted his work liberally in the first two *NROL* books, and if anything, he's become even more influential since then.

McGill says this in *Low Back Disorders*, his landmark textbook: "Enough sit-ups will cause damage in most people."

This is intensely counterintuitive, since the sit-up has a long history not just as an exercise to train abdominal muscles, but as the main way we measure their strength and endurance. (See "This Is Only a Test," page 6.) If we shouldn't do sit-ups, what should we do? Crunches? Reverse crunches? Leg raises? Actually, no. Despite the fact that they appeared in the first two *NROL* books, Alwyn's current workout programs don't include any exercises that force you to bend the spine to contract your abdominal muscles.

Why? Two reasons:

First, in the view of Alwyn and a growing number of strength and conditioning professionals, spine-bending exercises come up short when you calculate risk versus reward. There's not enough benefit to justify the potential risk to your lower back.

Second—and far more important—is that we've found better exercises to replace the crunches and leg raises. As I'll explain in great detail in the next few chapters, these exercises develop strength, stability, and endurance in your mid-body muscles without putting your spine at risk.

NEW RULE #3 • The size of your abdominal muscles doesn't matter.

I don't think anybody walks into the gym thinking, "Today I'm going to do whatever it takes to make my abs bigger." But sit-ups, leg raises, and crunches—the exercises you *won't* see in *NROL for Abs*—target your abdominal muscles directly for just that reason: to make them bigger and stronger. That's especially true of exercises like weighted sit-ups and crunches, hanging leg raises, and kneeling cable crunches.

Suppose you add size and strength to your midsection. What have you actually accomplished? Here's what McGill says in *Low Back Disorders*: "Several studies have shown that muscle strength cannot predict who will have future back troubles."

What matters is the *stability* those muscles provide, their ability to keep your spine in a safe position. To put it another way, *lack* of stability is a pretty strong predictor of who'll get lower-back injuries. Among female athletes, for example, problems with core stability can even predict knee injuries.

Size does matter when it comes to muscle atrophy—that is, if your muscles shrink due to injury or disuse, your core stability will suffer. But there doesn't seem to be a compelling argument that making those muscles bigger gives you more stability.

This Is Only a Test

In a 2001 study published in *Medicine & Science in Sports & Exercise*, researchers found that sit-up performance, more than any other measure of muscular fitness, was linked to longevity. They tested more than eight thousand men and women between the ages of twenty and sixty-nine, and then tracked them for the next twelve years. The ones who could do the fewest sit-ups were more than twice as likely to die during the thirteen-year follow-up period as the ones who could do the most.

They also measured push-up performance, handgrip strength, and flexibility, but none of those could be associated with a longer life.

The sit-up test, like the push-up test, is mostly a measure of muscular endurance, rather than strength. If you work your way up from five to ten repetitions, you've increased your strength. But if you go from forty to sixty reps, that's a sign of improved endurance. And in this study, endurance on sit-ups clearly trumped endurance on push-ups.

Now, suppose for a moment that this study had stumbled on the one true secret to longer life. Wouldn't we advise you to start doing sit-ups, despite the risk of injury to your lower back?

The U.S. Army conducted a study on this very topic; it was published in late 2009. The researchers had one group of soldiers train for their physical-fitness test the traditional way, with workouts that included sit-ups. Which makes sense, considering that the test requires soldiers to complete as many sit-ups as possible in two minutes. Another group trained with a nontraditional mix of core-stabilization exercises, with no sit-ups.

The study reports no significant differences between the two groups on their fitness tests after twelve weeks of training. Moreover, there was no statistically meaningful difference in *sit-up performance*. By developing the stability of the core muscles, the soldiers demonstrated improvements in core endurance.

So, to answer my own question, no, we probably wouldn't include sit-ups in the program.

NEW RULE #4 • The appearance of your midsection doesn't matter either.

During the twelve years I worked at *Men's Fitness* and *Men's Health* magazines, I supervised hundreds of photo shoots with models who rocked the lean, muscular, athletic physiques sought by our readers. However you want to describe their abs— "ripped," "quilted," "like giant raviolis"—these guys had 'em. But despite the uniform appearance, there was absolutely no way to predict which models could do the exercises with good form and which ones couldn't.

Some were amazing athletes, strong and well-coordinated guys whose performance in the gym matched their appearance. But some couldn't do basic exercises like squats and deadlifts. A few were so inflexible they couldn't touch their toes, never mind performing the more sophisticated and advanced core-training exercises.

Worst of all were the guys who'd gone on radical fat-reduction programs to get lean for the shoot. Readers would've been shocked to see how weak these guys were, how their arms and legs shook as they tried to hold their bodies in position long enough for the photographer to focus the camera and click off some shots. (This was back in the predigital days, when we shot entire rolls of film for each exercise.)

Of course one of our major goals in *NROL for Abs* is to help you develop a lean, contoured midsection. That's why we have so many chapters on nutrition and lifestyle modifications to help you gain muscle and lose fat. But we want you to understand up front that you can develop a strong, stable, healthy core even if you don't end up with abs like a cover model. Conversely, as I've witnessed many times, it's entirely possible to develop cover-model abs despite having a weak, dysfunctional core.

The best possible outcome is to have both a healthy core and strong abs. And the second-best outcome is to have great core stability and strength with an overall physique that still needs some work. Function is far more important than appearance.

ARGUMENTS WITH OURSELVES

Alwyn and I published *The New Rules of Lifting for Women* in January 2008. Not long after that, a potential client visited Results Fitness, Alwyn's gym in Southern California. She went through a trial workout, but didn't return. When the gym's manager called to ask why she'd changed her mind, she told him it was because she was reading our book. "You guys are almost there," she said, "but you don't completely get it yet."

Obviously, Alwyn and the trainers at his gym get it. But "it" is a moving target. Thousands of studies are published each year in the major exercise-science journals, and practitioners write thousands of articles about training and nutrition in magazines and online. We wouldn't be doing our jobs if we ignored new information, and we wouldn't be serving our readers if we chose consistency over adaptation.

As Alwyn likes to say, just because we changed our minds doesn't mean we were wrong before. It means we've refined our approach based on better information.

We've had to adapt a lot since 2006, when the original *New Rules of Lifting* came out—me because of the way my body changed with my series of unfortunate events, Alwyn because of the ways his clientele evolved in reaction to busier lives and smaller keyboards and screens.

The basics haven't really changed, but our application of the basics has.

Nowhere is that more pronounced than in our approach to training the core, the muscles that attach to your hips, pelvis, and lower back. Most of the rules we presented in the first two *NROL* books apply equally well to core training. (You can find a complete list of the rules in the Appendix on pages 257–259.) But we apply some of them in different ways than we did just a few years ago.

Take the first rule in the original *NROL*: "The best muscle-building exercises are the ones that use your muscles the way they're designed to work."

The only way this rule allows for an evolving application is if our understanding of functional anatomy evolves, which is exactly what happened with core training. That's why the workouts in *NROL for Abs* don't include crunches, hanging leg raises, Russian twists, and other exercises that appeared in one or both of the first two *NROL* books.

But as important as our new approach to core training is, I think the other changes to Alwyn's workout system are every bit as crucial.

- Increased mobility, especially in combination with better core strength and stability, helps you feel better every waking hour. (You might also feel better when you're asleep, but it's hard to assess such things unless you're awake.)
- You'll be doing less total strength training, but you may get more out of your workouts than you have in the past. The extra time you spend on mobility and core training will wake up and activate your muscles before you challenge them in the weight room. I can't say if this translates to more muscle fibers used per lift or more calories burned. All I can say is that it seems to work that way for Alwyn's clients.

- Starting with Phase Two of the three-stage program, the final ten to twenty minutes of each workout are devoted to metabolic work—high-effort, high-reward circuits of exercises that improve your conditioning and burn calories as fast as they can be burned. You'll get leaner, of course, but you'll also improve your ability to work hard inside or outside the gym.

But before I get into those details, let's talk about something more fundamental: What the heck is the core, anyway?

Core Curriculum

BEFORE WE CAN TALK ABOUT how to develop the core, we have to decide what the core is. I threw around a bunch of terms in the first chapter—"stability," "strength," "[abs] like giant raviolis"—but it's all just jargon unless we map out our territory.

Let's start with the big idea, and then work our way down. Don't worry if you don't recognize the names of some muscles on first reference; I'll explain each of them as we go along.

NEW RULE #5: • **The core includes all the muscles that attach to your hips, pelvis, and lower back.**

This list includes all the muscles you were thinking about when you bought this book . . .

- the four layers of the abdominals (rectus abdominis, external and internal obliques, transverse abdominis)
- hip flexors

- hip extensors (hamstrings, gluteals)
- spine extensors (spinal erectors, quadratus lumborum)
- hip adductors (inner-thigh muscles)
- hip abductors (including gluteus medius)
- multifidus (a muscle you never hear about until you have back pain)

. . . and one you probably hadn't considered:

NEW RULE #6 • The lats are part of the core.

The main job of the latissimus dorsi—the pair of fan-shaped muscles on the sides of your back—is to pull your arms downward. Hence, the "lat pulldown" uses your lats to pull a bar down toward your chest. Or, in the case of a pull-up or chin-up, you use the muscles to pull your chest up toward a bar. Your lats are crucial in any activity that involves climbing, pulling, or rowing.

But they also play a surprising role in stabilizing your spine and pelvis.

When we talk about muscles in technical terms, we look at "origins" and "insertions." Most of the time a muscle pulls a bone from the muscle's point or points of insertion toward its origin, which is usually the part that's closest to the body's midline. The easiest way to visualize this is to think of a simple muscle, like the biceps. It pulls the bones of your forearms (insertion) toward your shoulder (origin).

Your lats have relatively small points of insertion on your upper-arm bones. But the origins extend from your thoracic spine (middle back) to the top of your pelvis; some of the connective tissues in between reach all the way down to your tailbone. With so many points of origin, distributed so widely, the muscles have to pull double duty: They work to stabilize your spine, even as they're acting as prime movers for your upper arms.

Imagine yourself rock climbing. You reach up, grab a ledge, and pull with your left hand, while simultaneously pushing off another part of the rock wall with your right leg. As you rise, you reach for a new toehold with your left foot, and pray that your right hand lands on something solid. Your lats allow you to pull with your left hand, and your glute and thigh muscles generate the force to push with your right foot. But what's in between? Well, everything I listed earlier. But even with all those movers and stabilizers, you still need those connective tissues from your latissimus dorsi to help your lower back remain in a stable position.

So many muscles, so many actions. We'll start with the smallest and deepest, and work our way out.

THE LITTLE GUYS

When we talk about stability, what we really mean is that we want the lower back—the lumbar spine—to move as little as possible when it faces a challenge. This small range of movement is called the *neutral zone.* The smaller and tighter it is, the more stability you have.

Any number of conditions or events could expand the neutral zone and make your spine less stable:

- injury
- arthritis
- weakness in key muscles
- unbalanced strength among several muscles responsible for opposing movement patterns
- poor coordination among the core muscles
- muscles that simply don't work the way they're supposed to

As an example of the latter, McGill and others use the phrase "gluteal amnesia" to describe a condition in which athletes can't fully activate one or both sides of their gluteus maximus. It sounds funny until you consider that the work the glutes can't do is transferred to back muscles that aren't prepared to handle it. This creates the paradox of a really strong back that's more vulnerable to injury because the only reason it got so strong is the dysfunction of the glutes. The strength of the back masks the weakness of the glutes until it's too late.

So what keeps your spine in that neutral zone?

It starts with the twin *multifidus* muscles, which run up the sides of your spine. No other muscles are as deeply and intimately involved in the defense of your neutral zone. Multifidi provide stability to each individual segment of your lumbar spine, helping to control both rotation and backward bending.

The deepest abdominal layer, the *transverse abdominis* (TA), creates stability in a completely different way. Whereas the multifidi run north and south, the fibers of the TA go east and west. The muscle compresses your internal organs, and the pressure helps secure your spine in a stable position.

Unless you have an injury, the actions of these two muscles are automatic; your brain activates them to stabilize your spine before you move anything else.

The next-deepest abdominal muscles are the *internal obliques.* Like the TA, the internal obliques contribute compressive forces to help stabilize the spine. Their connective tissues merge with those of the lats to form a belt-like protective mechanism in your lower back.

The TA, multifidi, and internal obliques are mostly made up of slow-twitch muscle fibers. These are endurance-oriented muscles, designed to go long rather than generate a lot of power in a short burst. That's why the internal obliques are considered especially important for maintaining good posture. They can produce small amounts of force for a long time.

That said, the internal obliques are also involved in some power movements, working with your bigger, stronger abdominal muscles to flex your torso forward, bend to the side, or twist . . . or to resist any of those movements.

THE MOVERS AND SHAKERS

The *quadratus lumborum* is a small but important muscle in your lower back. You have one on each side, with origins on the top of your pelvis and insertions on your bottom rib and the vertebrae of your lumbar spine. Now, with insertions that are closer to the midline of your body than its origins, you can guess that one of its roles is to pull your torso to the side. The quadratus on your left side can pull you to the left, while the one on the right can straighten you back up again.

So when you see people doing side bends in the gym, they're strengthening their quadratus lumborum, along with their obliques.

But in real life, how often do you need to bend or straighten your body against some form of resistance? Not often, right? Thus, the main job of the quadratus muscles is to prevent bending movements that would take your spine out of its neutral zone.

The quadratus muscles also help in what's called *spinal extension*, which means straightening your back when it's bent forward. But their role in extension is minor compared to that of the *spinal erectors*, the muscles that run up the sides of your spine. When you've spent a lot of time around shirtless male fitness models, like I have, you can tell in an instant which ones are serious lifters. They have muscles like twin pythons running up the middle of their backs.

It's easy to see why these muscles get so thick and strong in male powerlifters. Imagine lifting from the floor a barbell that's two or three times your body's weight. The actual movement of your lumbar vertebrae is very small, just a few degrees. But the effort it takes to *prevent* spinal movement is mind-boggling. So even though the power to pull that weight off the floor comes mostly from your glutes and hamstrings, the strength to keep your spine in its neutral zone comes from your spinal erectors.

The next big-time midsection movers are your *external obliques*. From their position on the sides of your waist, they provide movement by allowing you to bend and twist, and provide stability by helping you resist those same movements.

You could say the same thing about the *rectus abdominis*, the much-obsessed-over six-pack muscle on the front of your abdomen. It contracts powerfully during a crunch—a movement called *spinal flexion*—along with the external obliques. That's why Alwyn used crunches in the first two *NROL* books. But we now know that it works even harder in exercises in which you resist spinal movement.

A few paragraphs ago, I noted that the spinal erectors get bigger and stronger when you do exercises like the deadlift, in which they're fighting to prevent your spine from going into flexion—a forward bend in which you flatten out your back's normal arch. The rectus abdominis, it turns out, works hardest when it resists a challenge that would put the spine into extension—a backward bend.

Two key studies changed Alwyn's mind about using crunches in his workouts. In the first, which came out in 2006, researchers compared the basic crunch and sit-up to exercises performed on a bunch of devices pushed on the public via infomercials—Ab Rocker, Torso Track, Ab Doer, and so on.

The big winners were the Ab Slide and Torso Track, machines that force you to extend your body while keeping your back in a safe, neutral position. Have you ever seen people in your gym doing rollout exercises with those little wheels that have handles on the sides? Exact same thing. The study showed that muscle activation of the rectus abdominis was about 30 percent higher on rollouts than it was on the standard crunch.

Another study, published in 2008, found that the two exercises were closer in total muscle activation, but the rectus abdominis still worked about 25 percent harder on the Ab Slide than it did on the crunch.

That's why Alwyn's workouts in *NROL for Abs* use walkout- and rollout-type exercises instead of crunches to work your primary abdominal muscles. Not only are they safer for your back, they're also more effective.

THE MISUNDERSTOOD MIDDLE MANAGERS

In my formative years as a fitness writer, the two scariest words were "hip flexors." As in, "If you do an exercise that involves your hip flexors, you'll hurt your back."

I found this perplexing. Hip flexors perform an action called *hip flexion*—lifting your leg in front of your body. You can't run or climb without using your hip flexors. They're important muscles, and it was hard for me to understand the problem with making them stronger. I still went along with all the wise men and women in my field, who said we had to stop doing full sit-ups because they rely too much on hip-flexor action. I dutifully told readers to do crunches instead of sit-ups. But I was never completely sold on the program.

I understand now that the concern was over one particular set of hip flexors, called the *psoas*. In concert with another muscle, the *iliacus*, they're the only muscles that can lift your thighs above 90 degrees. Because the psoas connect the thigh to the lumbar spine, they're capable of pulling your lower back out of its neutral position if they exert too much force, or if the force they exert isn't countered by equally strong muscles.

But here's why you can't ignore your hip flexors: Modern life requires hours of sitting with our thighs flexed to about 90 degrees, which over time shortens the muscles. Shortened hip flexors pull the top of the pelvis forward, drawing your

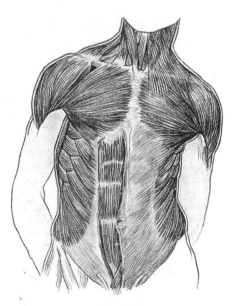

lower back into a more pronounced arch. In other words, doing nothing for your hip flexors produces the same result as using them too much in ill-advised exercises. Either way, you put your lower back at risk.

Alwyn's workouts include a mix of exercises that stretch and strengthen these often-neglected muscles. But your best defense against hip-flexor malfunction is to move around more during the day, a topic I'll explore in Chapter 13.

Two other sets of muscles that get little respect, especially in workout programs designed for guys, are the *hip adductors* and *hip abductors*. The adductors are inner-thigh muscles, which (big surprise!) pull your thighs inward. You can guess that the ab-

Hip Check

Here are two quick and fun tests, courtesy of our friend Mike Boyle, to see if you have properly functioning hip flexors:

First, stand on your left foot and pull your right knee to your chest. Let go. You should be able to keep your thigh above 90 degrees of flexion for at least 10 to 15 seconds. Repeat with the other leg.

Second, place one foot on a bench or step that's about 24 inches high. You want your thigh to be above 90 degrees of flexion—beyond parallel to the floor, in other words. With your hands above or behind your head, lift that foot off the bench. You should be able to hold it in the air for at least 5 seconds. Repeat with the other leg.

If you can't pass either test, or you have to bend or twist or otherwise distort your posture to pull it off, your hip flexors aren't as strong as they should be.

ductors do the opposite, lifting your thighs out and away from the midline of your body. The main abductor is the *gluteus medius*, which is on the side of your hip. These muscles get a workout when you do single-leg versions of exercises like squats and deadlifts. They have a big role in maintaining hip and pelvis stability, which affects the mechanics of everything from your torso down to your feet.

THE POWER BROKERS

The *gluteus maximus* is, or at least should be, your body's strongest muscle. It combines with your *hamstrings* to perform an action called *hip extension,* which is the source of almost all your athletic power. Your hip extensors get you off the ground when you jump, propel you forward when you sprint, and provide the pure strength that allows you to lift an empty sofa or a loaded barbell off the floor. (Or a loaded sofa, if those distant relatives *just won't take the hint* that it's time to leave.)

I mentioned earlier that the smaller muscles of

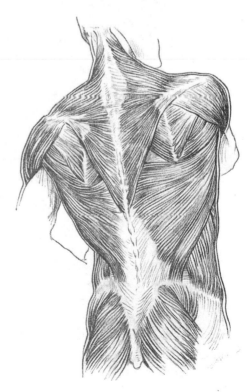

your abdomen and lower back consist mostly of slow-twitch muscle fibers, the ones capable of generating low levels of force for extended periods of time. So if we need endurance-oriented muscles to provide core stability, how do power-oriented muscles like the glutes and hamstrings fit into the picture?

Two ways.

First, when those muscles are strong and functional, your spine has more protection within its neutral zone. The spinal erectors can do their job, keeping your spine from bending forward, without having to overcompensate by bending your spine backward, distorting your posture in the opposite direction.

Second, if you look at an anatomy chart showing the human physique from the back, you'll see something interesting: The fibers of the lats on the left side of your

Gaga for Glutes?

For the past decade or so, I've heard various strength coaches and lecturers suggest that core training is almost entirely unnecessary. If you merely train hard enough with exercises like deadlifts and squats, there's no need to do specific exercises for your abdominal muscles. No other exercise could match the powerful torso-bracing contractions of your core muscles on those basic lifts.

In other words, train your glutes for strength and power, and everything else develops proportional strength and stability.

It's an interesting hypothesis, but it's been invalidated by at least two studies I know of. Back in 1998, researchers (including McGill) tested core-muscle activation on a couple dozen activities, ranging from sitting and standing to sit-ups and deadlifts with as much as 220 pounds. The abdominal muscles registered hardly any activity on the heavy deadlift. By comparison, the rectus abdominis and external obliques were far more active on basic push-ups.

Eight years later, Jeff McBride, an exercise scientist at Appalachian State University, tried something similar. He monitored muscle activation of experienced lifters who were using as much as 90 percent of their one-repetition maximum on squats and deadlifts. Once again, the abdominal muscles were far more active on push-ups than they were on even the heaviest squats and deadlifts.

McBride had the lifters do push-ups with their feet on a Swiss ball, which is much more of a challenge to core stabilizers. So this isn't an apples-to-apples comparison with the earlier study. But the results are similar enough to conclude that you can't train all your core muscles with one or two exercises.

body seem to run straight into the fibers of the gluteus maximus on your right. The two muscles form a series of diagonal lines from the armpit on one side to the outer hip on the other.

And what's in between? Your lower back. It's at the intersection of the fibers that run from your left lat to your right glute, and from your right lat to your left glute.

The No-Crunch Zone

When I first became a certified personal trainer, back in the mid-1990s, the functions of the major abdominal muscles were clear and uncontroversial: Bend the trunk forward or sideways. If you wanted to target those muscles, according to the textbook I studied to pass the test, the "selected exercises" included "bent-knee sit-ups," "partial curl-ups," "twisting bent-knee sit-ups," and "good posture."

Yes, the abdominal muscles do all those things, which is why sit-ups, crunches, and their twisting variations have been the ab-training exercises of choice for generations. But are those the functions those muscles *should* perform, or merely actions they *can* perform?

This is one of the most difficult and counterintuitive arguments to make with veteran gym rats. How do you explain to someone who's been doing crunches for ten or twenty years, or whose coach or personal trainer told them to do crunches, that it's a poor exercise choice for today's lifters?

I'll start with that challenge, and then move on to the most important information you'll find in this book: Alwyn's core-training system.

NEW RULE #7 • The crunch is not a core exercise.

It's an "ab" exercise, in that it works the rectus abdominis and obliques through a range of motion. To almost everyone who exercises, in or out of a gym, the crunch is to the abs as the biceps curl is to the biceps.

I'm no fan of the biceps curl, but I'm not foolish enough to suggest it doesn't help you build bigger arms, which is of course the entire point. The crunch probably increases the size of your rectus abdominis and obliques as well, if you make it challenging enough. The fibers in those muscles certainly have some potential for growth, and there's nothing wrong with having bigger, stronger muscles anywhere on your body.

But few of us crunch with the same intensity we devote to our curls. If your goal is to build your biceps, you'll probably do sets of curls with no more than eight to twelve repetitions, and you'll probably push yourself close to momentary muscular failure—the point when you can't do any more reps with that weight on that exercise.

Can you remember the last time you saw anyone perform crunches with that level of intensity? I can't. It would require using an external load, like a weight plate on the chest or behind the head, and continuing the set to the point of muscular exhaustion. A typical person in a typical health club will knock out a couple dozen reps with no external load, then maybe rest and repeat, or go on to another type of crunch.

What, exactly, are you training when you crunch like that, doing high-rep sets of a low-intensity exercise, and stopping well short of muscular failure? Honestly, I don't think you're training anything. You're reminding your muscles how to do a crunch, and you're probably preventing a loss of strength or muscle mass in your abdomen. But are you developing anything? Certainly not strength. Certainly not muscle size. And you sure as hell aren't developing core stability, because forcing your spine into flexion is the opposite of keeping it inside its neutral zone.

So you're flexing your spine for the sake of flexing your spine. Is that bad? Yes, because . . .

NEW RULE #8 • Your spine is already flexed, and flexing it more just makes it worse.

In a movie called *Miami Blues*, which came out in 1990, a cop played by Fred Ward has dinner with an ex-convict, who's played by Alec Baldwin. He knows the man is an ex-con because of the way he eats, hunching over his food as if to guard it from his fellow inmates. I thought about that scene not long ago when I was in a family restaurant with my wife and kids. After nagging my children to sit up straight and get their elbows off the table, I looked around and noticed that virtually everyone else in the restaurant—parents as well as children—was hunched forward over their food, leaning on their forearms for support. By *Miami Blues* standards, they all looked like ex-cons.

Why are all these people hunched over? Have table manners changed so dramatically in a single generation? Or have the people at the tables changed?

I noted in the Introduction that Alwyn's new clients are physically less fit than demographically identical clients just a few years ago. They come in with more body

Punch-Drunk Abs

At this point in the book, you may be formulating a counterargument: If spinal flexion is so bad, why do we have such interesting-looking muscles capable of performing it?

I was curious about that as well, and found an answer in *Anatomy Trains*, a book for physical therapists written by Thomas Myers. Humans, Myers writes, are the only animals with all our vulnerable parts—face, throat, viscera, genitals—right up in front of our bodies. (We have less vulnerability from the back, suggesting that as a species we're uniquely evolved to run away from our enemies.) Moreover, we have no special tools to defend ourselves from a frontal attack. We have no talons or natural armor, and our teeth are designed to chew food, rather than kill it.

My best guess is that this is an evolutionary accident. We started walking upright millions of years ago to conserve energy as we searched for food; chimps, by contrast, use far more energy to move the same distance as humans. That's how once-protected body parts became exposed and vulnerable. Apes, if attacked, are much better equipped to defend themselves, with bigger teeth, longer arms, and strength that surpasses ours by several orders of magnitude.

Back to those abdominal muscles: When we're attacked, or think we're going to be attacked, what do we do? We hunch. We contract our abs and roll our shoulders and arms forward, simultaneously tightening the sheath that protects our organs and using our arms to deflect a strike. Our chin drops to protect our throat. And if we think something might hit our genitals, we instinctively contract our inner-thigh muscles and lift a leg to guard the area.

One more point: Which athletes most need to train for spinal-flexion strength? Fighters. In MMA, you'll see a move called the clinch, in which one fighter grabs the back of his opponent's head and tries to pull it down to break his posture. Both fighters need extraordinary strength in their abdominal muscles—one to flex his spine, the other to keep his spine from being flexed.

Thus, if you're a fighter or an athlete in a contact sport—categories that include soldiers, martial artists, and football players—you need to work on spinal-flexion strength. If you're a gym rat, you don't need to worry about it.

fat (about 50 percent more, on average), worse balance and coordination (they usually have major discrepancies between the left and right sides of their bodies), and worse posture.

For now, let's focus on the latter. If you hunch over a laptop all day at the office, and use your lunch and dinner time to thumb out text messages and e-mails on your BlackBerry, and spend much of the rest of your day slumped forward or backward on a car seat, desk chair, or sofa, what will that do to your posture? You'll end up with a permanent slump, right? Your lower back will be flat, and your shoulders will roll forward.

In other words, your spine is constantly flexed. And if your spine is in that position anyway, why would you go into the gym and exacerbate the problem with set after set of a spine-flexing exercise like the crunch?

THE THREE CATEGORIES OF CORE EXERCISES

Now that I've told you what you *won't* be doing in the *NROL for Abs* workouts, let's look at what you will do. Alwyn's system features three basic categories of core exercises:

Stabilization

Another way to describe most of the exercises in this category is to say they develop *static stability*. That is, you put your body into a position in which you must stabilize your spine and pelvis, and hold it there for a designated amount of time. The most basic examples are the planks and side planks you've seen in *NROL for Women* . . . and just about every other forward-thinking book or article that includes core training. In the plank, you get into a prone position on the floor and balance your weight on your forearms and toes, with your body forming a straight line from your neck through your ankles.

That's the entry-level version of the exercise, and for some of you, it'll be challenging enough. Others will need to move up to more advanced variations in subsequent workouts. You must be able to hold the position for the prescribed amount of time before you move up.

The progressions, which you'll see illustrated and described in Chapter 5, work like this:

1. PLANK

Your goal here is to coordinate your deepest stabilizing muscles so they can hold a single position against the forces of gravity. You'll develop endurance in those muscles as you increase the amount of time they have to hold the position.

2. PLANK WITH SINGLE-ARM OR SINGLE-LEG SUPPORT

When you lift one arm or one leg off the floor, you've shifted your center of gravity, which offers a real and perhaps even dramatic challenge to your deep stabilizing muscles. The challenge from gravity is now asymmetrical, requiring a different strategy for coordinating those muscles, and requiring more strength on the side that's lost one of its support structures.

You'll also introduce a very basic dynamic component at this stage, since you'll be changing the leg or arm that's elevated while keeping your spine in its neutral zone.

In the most advanced variation at this level, you'll lift one arm and the opposite-side leg simultaneously, giving you just two points of support.

3. STABILIZATION ON AN UNSTABLE SURFACE

If you rest your hands or forearms on something that might move, like a Swiss ball, you introduce a systemic challenge to your core stability. This is more than an up-or-down battle against gravity. The ball can and will roll in any direction—left, right, forward, backward, or anywhere in between—and each time it does your core muscles have to make an adjustment to keep your lower back in its neutral zone, not to mention prevent you from falling over.

The first progression from the basic position, with four points of support, is to lift one leg and force your body to adjust to having just three contacts with the surface.

Next you'll elevate your feet onto a box or bench, which forces you to work harder against gravity. If you advance to the next progression (not everyone will), you'll lift one leg off the elevated surface. That gives you two hands or forearms on the ball, one foot on a box or bench, and the other foot in the air. Even the most advanced readers will find that one difficult.

Dynamic stabilization

In the static-stabilization category, most of the exercises require your deepest core muscles to generate low levels of force for increasing amounts of time. You're focusing primarily on slow-twitch muscle fibers, developing endurance that's critical for the safe performance of everything from sports to heavy lifting to yard work and home repair.

The dynamic-stabilization exercises, in which you're moving one or more limbs while keeping your spine in its neutral zone, bring more fast-twitch muscle fibers into the mix. Some of your core muscles will generate high levels of force relative to their size and functions.

The rollout-type exercises, which I mentioned in Chapter 2, are probably the best examples of dynamic stabilization. Typically, your feet are on the ground, with your hands resting on something that's moving forward, like a Swiss ball. The goal is to keep your spine in its neutral position while your center of gravity moves farther away from the middle of your body.

Another way to describe this category of exercises is to say they force you to stabilize *around* the core. The most basic stabilization exercises first teach you to coordinate the muscles that fix your lower back and pelvis in the neutral zone, and then to stay in the neutral zone as the challenges grow more complex. When you do dynamic-stabilization exercises, it's a given that the deepest core muscles are working hard to safeguard your spine within its neutral zone. The extra moving parts force other muscles to contribute.

Integrated stabilization

I've had to make a lot of adjustments to my workouts in recent years, thanks mostly to the series of injuries I described in the Introduction. To my surprise, many of them are improvements. One of my favorite exercises today is the one-arm dumbbell chest press, something I wouldn't have considered doing back in the days when I could knock out barbell bench presses without discomfort. If you saw someone doing it in a gym, you wouldn't think of it as a "core" exercise. It looks like it works the chest, shoulder, and triceps muscles on the side of the body that's holding the weight—which, of course, it does.

But when you actually try the exercise, and feel an intense contraction in your oblique muscles, you realize it's working a lot more than that. Because you're working one arm at a time, each set is really the equivalent of two sets, in terms of the amount of work you impose on your core muscles.

That's a perfect example of what we mean when we talk about integrated stabilization. To a casual observer, these exercises appear to target the prime movers—your pectoral muscles on a chest press, your upper-back muscles on a row, your legs on a squat or lunge variation. Nobody would guess that you're working your "core," never mind your "abs." But when you're doing the exercises, more often than not, you'll understand why they're included in a program designed to develop core strength and stability.

Which is not to say that they don't work the targeted muscles. As I sit here writing this section, my legs are sore as hell from yesterday's workout, which included high-rep sets of squats while holding a single weight at shoulder height. The exercise forced my core muscles to stabilize an unbalanced load—the weight of my torso plus the weight of a dumbbell on one side of it—while my legs were probably just lifting my body's weight plus the dumbbell, without having to make extraordinary accommodations for the fact that the weight threw off my center of gravity. I'm sure there was a difference in the way some of the smaller leg muscles worked to keep my body balanced, but I could feel the work being done by my quadriceps muscles while I was lifting, and I especially feel the soreness in those muscles today.

Most of the time, integrated-stabilization exercises won't work your muscles as hard as you could work them if you were doing the most straightforward versions of those exercises. On the squat, for example, you'll develop more size and strength using heavier weights held in front of or behind your shoulders. Same with the chest press I described earlier. If the goal is to build bigger pecs, shoulders, and arms, you'll make the biggest gains if you lie on your back on a bench and knock out presses with a barbell or two dumbbells.

Another way to say it: The most effective size- and strength-building exercises work your muscles within a single plane of motion. The more straightforward the exercise, the easier it is to work with heavy weights.

But that isn't the goal of integrated stabilization. You want your core muscles to learn to hold your spine in its neutral zone under conditions that most closely resemble what you'll encounter in sports and everyday life. When you're working in your garden, for example, almost all your heavy lifting is asymmetrical. You pick up a bag of mulch, throw it over one shoulder, and carry it wherever it needs to go. Even if you're carrying a load that appears symmetrical—imagine carrying a small child on your shoulders during a hike—in reality it's not that simple. Every time you take a step the load shifts slightly. The more uneven the ground, the more it shifts. And of course the kid himself is hardly sitting still. Every time he wriggles or turns to look at something or tries to grab something else, the challenge to your core muscles changes.

CATEGORICAL DENIAL

Now, having described the three categories of core-training exercises, I should note that they don't always represent progressive levels of difficulty. The most advanced variations in the stabilization category might be more difficult to perform than the integrated-stabilization exercises. They have fewer moving parts, but that's small consolation when you find yourself struggling to hold a static position that's completely novel to your muscles and nervous system.

Once you get to integrated stabilization, you'll no longer measure progress by the difficulty of the movement. You'll add weight, or reps, or distance, or even speed.

The cool thing is, you can repeat these programs any number of times and still find new ways to make progress. You'll always be getting better at something: strength, power, coordination, endurance. So each time you return to Alwyn's program, you'll be doing the exercises with a different body, or at least a body that's capable of a higher level of performance.

PART 2

FULL-SPECTRUM AB TRAINING

4

Drilling Down to the Core

You can look at the exercises shown in the next three chapters as just that— exercises. Some will draw stares, impress people at parties, or perhaps even scare small children. You can mix 'em, match 'em, trade 'em with your friends. But if you approach them as random movements to throw into a workout when you're bored, you'll get a small fraction of their benefits. Yes, you'll put your core muscles under tension for a designated amount of time, and of course there's value in that. You'll figure out if you have enough strength and skill for some of the trickier ones, and there's nothing wrong with testing yourself and pushing your limits.

Full value, however, comes with *progression*. First you master the stabilization exercises shown in Chapter 5. Then you move up to the dynamic-stabilization exercises shown in Chapter 6, and develop proficiency in those. Finally you tackle the integrated-stabilization moves in Chapter 7.

You also make progression within each category. The two most important stabilization exercises—plank and side plank—have multiple variations that offer increasing challenges in every aspect of fitness and efficacy. The exercises in the more advanced categories have fewer variations, but in most cases involve an external load—a weight to be lifted or balanced or otherwise accommodated. When there isn't an external load or more difficult variation, you make progress by increasing the speed of your repetitions. In every exercise, you want to advance as far as your time, ability, and ambition will allow you to go.

But you also want to start at the beginning.

The first time you do a new workout, choose the basic version of each exercise, or start with a relatively light weight, even if you're an experienced lifter. Do it for the maximum amount of time designated, or the maximum sets and reps. If it's easy, no problem. The next time you do that workout, choose a more advanced variation, or increase the resistance, or do it faster. Just make sure you've mastered the movement first—you can do it for the maximum amount of time or designated number of sets and reps, and you can do it with perfect form.

After you've maxed out the basic version, you choose how fast to progress, or how much additional resistance you want to use. You can move up slowly and incrementally until you reach a level at which the exercise is truly challenging. Or you can skip some steps if you're an experienced lifter and want to get to the tough stuff as soon as possible.

Just remember two important points:

- The time you spend at each level of the program is finite—just four to six weeks. So you don't want to make it too easy for too long, and pass up the opportunity to tackle more complex, interesting, and fun versions of the exercises.
- Conversely, you don't want to jump into the deep end unless you're absolutely sure you can swim back to the side.

I speak from experience on that second point. When I started the program I made the mistake of moving right up to the most challenging versions I thought I could do. Turns out, I couldn't get anywhere near the max on the ones I chose. I had to go through the progressions *backward* the next time I did those workouts.

If you're typically cautious in the gym, push yourself out of your comfort zone once you're familiar with the exercises. And if you're like me, and your first instinct is to skip ahead, try taking a more incremental approach. But no matter which end of the caution-ambition spectrum you find yourself on, or whether you're looking for security or novelty, there's plenty for everyone in the next three chapters.

THE THINGS YOU'LL CARRY

I'll acknowledge this right up front: The last thing you want to hear after you've just bought a fitness book is that you'll need to buy more stuff to do the workouts. Actually, there's only one workout tool that we strongly suggest purchasing. A couple things are nice to have, and the rest you should already own if you work out at home.

I'll start with the necessities.

VALSLIDES

Alwyn has been using these simple, inexpensive, and versatile workout tools with his clients for years. (You can see Alwyn's endorsement on the website valslides.com.) I bought my own set in 2008 after meeting their inventor, celebrity trainer Valerie Waters, at a seminar. I've carried them around in my gym bag ever since. For $35 plus shipping from performbetter.com, I consider them one of the best values to be found in fitness equipment.

Valslides have slick plastic on the bottom with a rubber grip on the top. You can hold them in your hands or set them under your feet. You'll use them once each way in Alwyn's workouts.

Can you do the workouts without buying your own set of slides? Yes. We show an alternative version of one of the exercises, and an alternative way to do the other. So purchasing or not purchasing is up to you.

SWISS BALL

Also called an exercise ball, physioball, or stability ball. I can't remember the last time I visited a gym that didn't have them. If you train at home, you should have one. (I have three, including one I've never taken out of the box, and I don't even work out at home.) They're a great tool for core training because they offer an unstable base of support, which forces your stabilizing muscles to work harder to keep your lower back and pelvis in their safe, neutral position. They're inexpensive, and you can buy one at any sporting-goods store.

BARBELL AND DUMBBELLS

For the strength exercises, you'll do best with an Olympic barbell set, in addition to a range of dumbbells (or one adjustable set). But for the core exercises, you just need dumbbells.

BOX AND BENCH

A sturdy six-inch box, or a pair of aerobics steps, will come in handy for several of the exercises. And a bench is absolutely necessary for the strength program. If you don't have them, you can pick them up at any sporting-goods store, or check out Craigslist for used equipment.

SUSPENSION TRAINERS

When Alwyn created the workouts for *NROL* and *NROL for Women*, this category of fitness equipment—straps that hang from a chin-up bar and allow you to suspend your hands or feet off the floor—barely existed. Now it's something Alwyn uses on a daily basis with his clients.

In the exercise descriptions, you'll see them described as "TRX or equivalent." TRX is the best-known and best-marketed brand in this category. They're also among the most expensive, starting at $150. Personally, I own a much cheaper trainer, called the Jungle Gym. It's just $40, and allows me to do all the same exercises, although it takes longer to get into or change positions. Want an even cheaper alternative? A couple of the biggest guys at my gym use a pair of dog leashes. As long as it's portable, holds your body weight, and allows you to attach it to something sturdy, it'll work.

You don't have to have a suspension trainer for these workouts—we give you plenty of alternatives in the next three chapters—but if you try them out, I think you'll like them. Once you've done a set of push-ups with your hands suspended, you may never go back to doing them on the floor.

You can find the TRX and Jungle Gym at performbetter.com. Blast Straps, another heavy-duty option, are available for $75 a pair at elitefts.com. For dog leashes, I'd start with Petco.

ELASTIC BANDS

If you don't have access to a cable machine, you'll need one of these—or more than one, if you want to create different levels of resistance. A thick band will also come in handy for the strength workouts. You can find them at performbetter.com or elitefts.com.

KETTLEBELLS

They look like a cannonball with a fixed handle. You can find them today in all shapes and sizes, from original cast iron to vinyl-coated and candy-colored. Their value as a training tool comes from the fact that the weight is offset. When you grip a dumbbell, the weight is at the same level as your hand. But when you hold a kettlebell, the weight is below the handle. That makes it an interesting and versatile tool for core training, as well as for power development and overall conditioning.

INTERVAL TIMER

You can use anything you want to clock yourself on the stability exercises that specify time instead of repetitions. If it has a second hand, it'll work. But I'll throw a plug in here for the Gymboss, a $20 interval timer designed specifically for people like us and workouts like these. It's one of my all-time favorite training toys. Check it out at gymboss.com.

Because of variations in strength, posture, training status, and athletic ability, no two individuals will perform each exercise with identical form. Readers should follow the written instructions as carefully as possible, and use the photos as a point of reference rather than as an instructional guide superseding the textual description of proper exercise form.

5

Stabilization

You'll see a lot of people in health clubs doing planks and side planks—no surprise, considering that these stabilization exercises have been a staple of workout books and fitness magazines since 2005 or thereabouts. But you'll almost never see anyone push him- or herself to do the more advanced variations shown and described on the following pages.

I think that's a mistake, although I understand how it happens. Most of the basic gym exercises—from frou-frou dumbbell kickbacks to hard-core squats and deadlifts—offer a simple and obvious way to make progress: Do more. More reps, more sets, more weight. But if someone told you to "do more" stabilization work, how would you comply? Would you do planks and side planks more often? Hold the positions longer?

Try it.

A few years back, I heard a trainer suggest that no one should do advanced ab-training exercises until he or she could hold a basic plank position for three minutes. Of course I took that as a challenge, and I started my next workout with a three-minute plank. To this day, I'm bitter about the experience. It was the most tedious three minutes of my life. Compared to 180 seconds of static stabilization, watching a Ken Burns documentary on PBS is an adrenaline rush.

If that's progression, no wonder so few people pursue it.

You, on the other hand, are in for a treat. For one thing, you'll never have to hold a plank for longer than 90 seconds—half that for a side plank. From there, you'll move up to exercises that are rarely seen in commercial health clubs. There's nothing boring about holding a plank in which your arms balance on a Swiss ball while your toes are up on a bench. I won't go so far as to say it's frightening, but it is precarious enough to keep you focused.

✳ Plank

GET READY

- If you don't have a well-padded, carpeted area to do this, find a mat and set it on the floor.
- Get into a modified push-up position, with your weight resting on your forearms and toes. Your forearms should be aligned with your torso, with your elbows directly beneath your shoulders.
- Your body should form a straight line from your neck through your ankles.

HOLD

- Hold that position for 60 to 90 seconds.

THINK

- Don't consciously flex any particular muscles. Let your body figure out how to keep your spine and pelvis in a neutral position.
- Pay attention to your muscles as the set goes on; you'll feel the bigger ones come into action as the smaller ones fatigue.

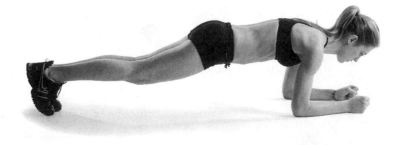

MODIFY

If you can't hold a plank at least 60 seconds, you can break up the set into smaller increments. Hold for as long as you can, rest for the exact amount of time that you held the position, and then repeat until you reach 60 seconds. In subsequent workouts, try to extend that initial hold by at least a few seconds each time you do the exercise.

DON'T . . .

- Lift your butt in the air, creating a hinge in your hips. It's no challenge at all to hold that position. If it weren't for the blood rushing to your head, you could stay there all day.
- Spread your feet wide apart. By increasing the base of support, you decrease the challenge to your core. (You will need to do this on some of the variations shown in the next few pages, but not on the basic plank.)

Alternative

✳ 45-Degree Plank

- If you have to do either of the modifications described above, you're not ready to start off with the traditional plank. Use this version to build strength and endurance.
- Rest your forearms on a padded exercise bench, and balance your weight on your forearms and toes.
- Align your body so it forms a straight line from your neck through your ankles.

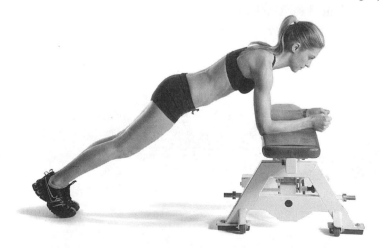

PLANK PROGRESSION SERIES #1: Reduced base of support

✳ Plank with Leg Lift

- From the plank position, lift one leg so the toes are at least a few inches off the floor.
- You can hold in that position for an entire set—60 to 90 seconds—and then do the second set with the other leg raised, or switch legs halfway through each set.

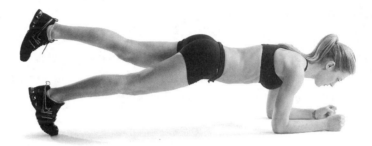

✳ Plank with Arm Lift

- You probably want to set up with your feet wider apart.
- Lift one arm out in front of or diagonal to your torso.
- Hold for 10 to 15 seconds, then switch arms, and continue for 60 to 90 seconds.
- This variation presents the first really big step up in difficulty. Doing a plank with one leg in the air isn't that much harder than the basic exercise, but as soon as you lift an arm off the floor you'll feel a complete shift in the way your core muscles work to balance your body.

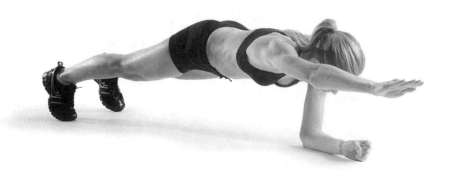

✳ Push-Up Hold with Arm Lift

- Get into the push-up position, with your hands directly below your shoulders. Make sure your body forms a straight line from your neck through your ankles.
- Spread your feet so they're wider than your shoulders.
- Lift one hand off the floor and extend it in front of you.
- Hold for 15 to 20 seconds, then switch arms.
- Start by lifting your dominant hand (your right if you're right-handed). When you switch and lift your nondominant arm, it should almost feel like you're taking a break.
- This variation on the plank with arm lift offers more of a full-body challenge, and probably works best for experienced lifters with well-developed upper-body strength.

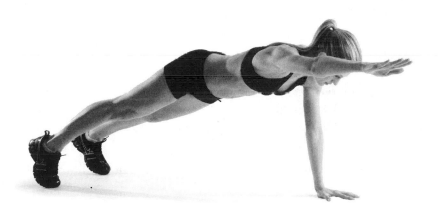

✳ Plank with Arm and Leg Lift

- From the plank position, lift one arm and the opposite-side leg.
- Hold for 5 to 15 seconds, then switch arms and legs.
- This is the second big step up in difficulty from the basic plank. It offers a simultaneous challenge to your core strength, stability, and endurance, as well as your balance and coordination.

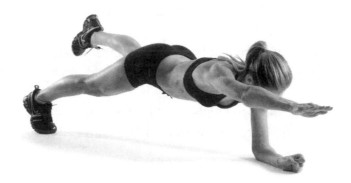

Alternative

✳ Push-Up Hold with Arm and Leg Lift

- Get into the push-up position with your hands beneath your shoulders and your feet wider than your shoulders.
- Lift one arm and the opposite-side leg.
- Hold for 10 to 15 seconds, then switch arms and legs.
- Similar to the push-up hold with arm lift, this variation will work best for those with advanced upper-body strength.

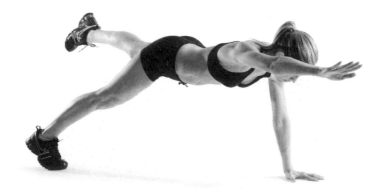

PLANK PROGRESSION SERIES #2: Unstable Support

✳ Swiss-Ball Plank

- Set up with your forearms on the Swiss ball and your toes on the floor.
- Your body should form a straight line from your neck through your ankles.
- Hold for 60 to 90 seconds.

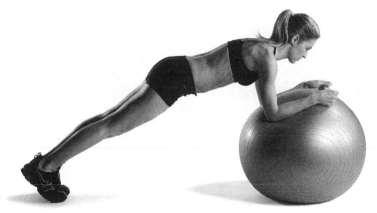

Alternative #1

✳ Swiss-Ball Push-Up Hold

- Set up with your hands on the Swiss ball and your toes on the floor.
- Hold for 60 to 90 seconds.

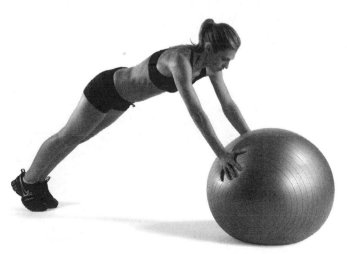

Alternative #2

✳ Suspended Push-Up Hold

- Attach a TRX or equivalent to a chin-up bar or something equally sturdy.
- Adjust the length to match your ability— the closer the handles are to the floor, the more difficult it should be.
- Grab the handles and suspend yourself in the push-up position, with your toes on the floor. Your body should form a straight line from your neck through your ankles.

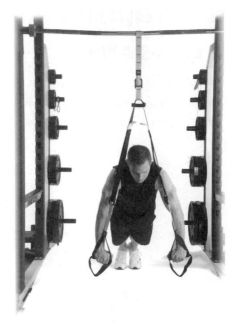

✳ Swiss-Ball Plank with Leg Lift

- From the plank position, lift one foot off the floor.
- You can hold that position for an entire set—60 to 90 seconds—and then do the second set with the other leg raised, or switch legs halfway through the set.
- Obviously, this is a progression within the progression, combining an unstable element with a reduced base of support.
- You can also add a leg lift to the Swiss-ball push-up hold or the suspended push-up hold.

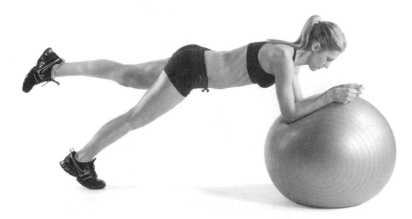

PLANK PROGRESSION SERIES #3: Feet elevated

✳ Plank with Feet Elevated

- Set up with your toes on a bench and your forearms on the floor.
- Your body should form a straight line from your neck through your ankles, which means your head will be angled downward slightly.
- Hold for 60 to 90 seconds.

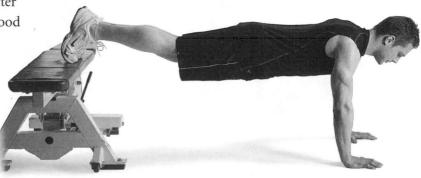

Important note: In Phase One, Workout B, you'll *start* with this exercise. Instead of holding for 60 to 90 seconds, you'll hold for 10 seconds, relax for a second or two, and repeat until you do a total of 10 holds. (The workout structure is explained in detail in Chapter 8, and you'll find the Phase One workouts in Chapter 10.)

Alternative

✳ Push-Up Hold with Feet Elevated

- Same exercise, but better suited to those with good upper-body strength.

✳ Plank with Feet Elevated and Leg or Arm Lift

- Set up as before, and raise one leg or one arm for 10 seconds.

- I don't know if it's just me, but raising a foot off the bench and holding it up seems to come close to the difficulty of raising an arm from the same position. When your toes are on the floor, as I noted earlier, it's much easier to raise one leg than it is to raise one arm.

- I know this is skipping ahead, but it'll make sense when you get into the gym and start working your way through the program: If you're doing Phase One, Workout B, in which you hold each position for 10 seconds, you can cycle through all four limbs. So you'd lift your right leg for 10 seconds, relax, lift your left leg, relax, right arm, left arm, repeat. You won't be able to do each limb the same number of times, but trust me: After 10 of these holds, you won't worry about it.

- We don't recommend trying to lift one arm and the opposite-side leg simultaneously in this progression. The angle seems to force your cervical (upper) spine out of alignment.

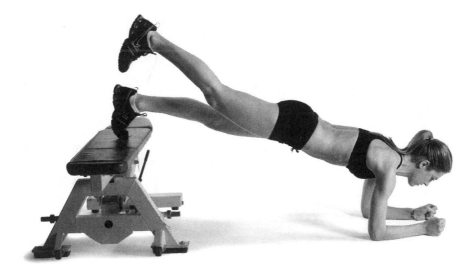

✳ Push-Up Hold with Feet Elevated + Leg or Arm Raise, Or Simultaneous Leg And Arm Raise

- Start with your hands below your shoulders, and do any or all of the variations described for the plank with feet elevated.
- If you're both strong and daring, you can do an arm raise with opposite-side leg raise from a push-up hold with your feet elevated. Your body is more or less parallel to the floor, so there's less risk of losing your spinal alignment.
- If you work up to this variation in Phase One, Workout B, raise your right arm and left foot, hold for 10 seconds, relax for a second or two, then repeat with your left arm and right leg elevated.

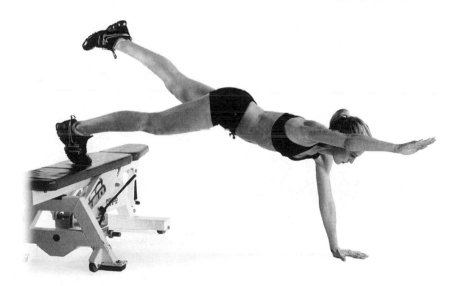

PLANK PROGRESSION SERIES #4: Feet elevated + unstable support

✳ Swiss-Ball Plank with Feet Elevated

- Set up with your forearms on the Swiss ball and your toes on the bench.
- Intermediate-level lifters may be able to do this variation in Workout B for 10 seconds at a time by the end of Phase One.
- Advanced lifters may be able to do this variation in Workout A for 60 to 90 seconds by the end of Phase One.

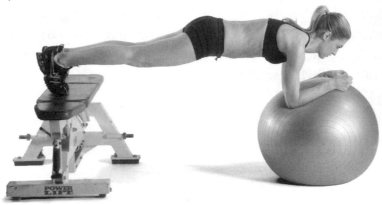

Alternative #1

✳ Push-Up Hold with Feet Elevated on Swiss Ball

- Set up with your hands on the floor, shoulder-width apart, and your toes on the Swiss ball.
- This is an interesting, challenging exercise that doesn't require as much upper-body strength as some of the other variations on the push-up hold. But it takes a lot of core strength and coordination, particularly in the muscles of the pelvis and inner thighs.
- Focus on alignment; with your feet higher than your shoulders and balanced on an unstable surface, your instinct will be to raise your hips. If you can't set up next to a mirror, ask a trainer or knowledgeable friend to check your form.

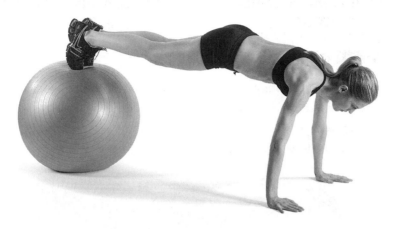

Alternative #2

✳ Suspended Push-Up Hold with Feet Elevated

- Set up the TRX or equivalent so your hands will be suspended roughly 18 to 36 inches off the floor.
- Set up a bench the appropriate distance from the suspension handles.
- Grab the handles and set your toes on the bench.
- Get into the push-up position with your body forming a straight line from your neck to your ankles, and hold.

Alternative #3

✳ Push-Up Hold with Feet Suspended

- Set up the TRX or equivalent so your feet will be suspended roughly 12 to 24 inches off the floor.
- Put your feet into the loops.
- Get into push-up position, and hold.

PLANK PROGRESSION SERIES #5: Feet elevated + unstable support + reduced base of support

✳ Swiss-Ball Plank with Feet Elevated + Leg Raise

- Set up with your forearms on the Swiss ball and toes on the bench.
- Raise one leg, hold for 10 seconds, lower it, and raise the other.
- Hats off to anyone who can hold this position 10 times for 10 seconds. And if you can hold it for 60 to 90 seconds, count me as one of your fans.

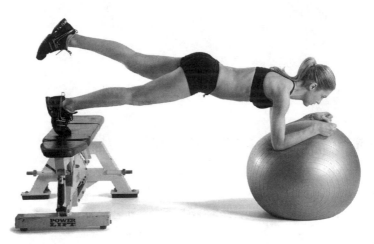

Alternative #1

✳ Push-Up Hold with Feet Elevated on Swiss Ball + Leg Raise

- Set up as described previously, then lift one foot off the ball for 10 seconds, lower it, and raise the other.
- This probably is less difficult than the previous exercise, the Swiss-ball plank with feet elevated + leg raise. To me, having your upper body on the unstable surface is more challenging.

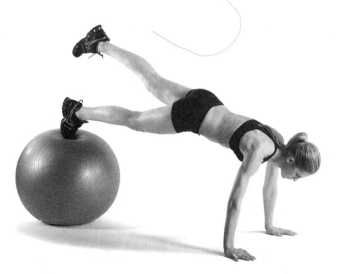

Alternative #2

✳ Suspended Push-Up Hold with Feet Elevated + Leg Raise

- Grab the handles of the TRX or equivalent, and rest your toes on the bench.
- Raise one leg, hold for 10 seconds, lower it, and raise the other.
- Yes, this is the most challenging exercise in the plank series.

✳ Side Plank

GET READY

- Even if you're working out on a carpeted floor with good padding beneath it, you'll probably want to use a mat to rest your forearm. And if you're doing this on a hard surface, I recommend using two mats. Much of your body weight will be resting on your elbow and forearm, and you need the extra protection.

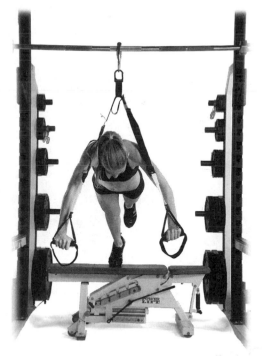

- Lie on your left side with your legs straight and your right leg on top of your left.
- Position yourself so your weight is resting on your left forearm and the outside edge of your left foot. Your elbow should be directly beneath your shoulder, and your upper arm should be perpendicular to the floor.
- Align your body so it forms a straight line from your neck to your ankles.
- You can place your right hand on your left shoulder or on your right hip, whichever works better for you.

HOLD

- Hold that position for 30 to 45 seconds.
- Relax, switch sides, and repeat.

THINK

- "Long." As in, an elongated torso. You'll feel the exercise in the oblique muscles on the side closest to the floor, but if you consciously think about those muscles flexing, you'll shorten your torso and lose your alignment.
- You want to keep your shoulders square and on a plane that's perpendicular to the floor. Imagine that they're pressed against a wall behind you.

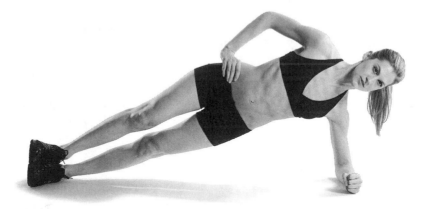

MODIFY

If you can't hold a side plank for at least 30 seconds, you can break up the set into smaller increments. Hold for as long as you can, rest for the exact amount of time that you held the position, and then repeat until you reach 30 seconds. In subsequent workouts, try to extend that initial hold by at least a few seconds each time you do the exercise.

DON'T . . .

- Allow your hips to sag toward the floor. This changes your posture from a straight line to a boomerang.
- Crunch your abs. By pulling the rectus abdominis into the movement, you rotate your torso and bring your top shoulder toward the floor. If you think this is happening, you can do the side plank with your back against a wall. If you lose contact with the wall, you know your torso has started to rotate.

Alternative

✳ Modified Side Plank

- If you can't hold the side plank for even a few seconds, you'll have to build a base of core strength and endurance with this version.
- Bend your knees, so your weight rests on your left forearm and the outside edge of your left knee.
- Align your body so it forms a straight line from your neck through your knees.
- Transition away from the modified side plank as soon as you can. You're

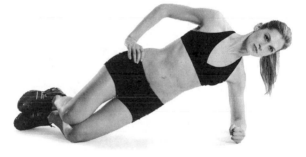

only supporting a fraction of your body weight, which compromises the potential benefits. It's better to do the traditional side plank in limited time increments, and build up core strength and endurance over time.

SIDE PLANK PROGRESSION SERIES #1: Increased resistance

✳ Side Plank with Arm Overhead

- Instead of resting your right hand on your left shoulder or right hip, hold it overhead.
- Even though you're adding just a bit more gravitational pressure, this version is more challenging than you expect the first time you try it, especially when you try to hold for the full 45 seconds.

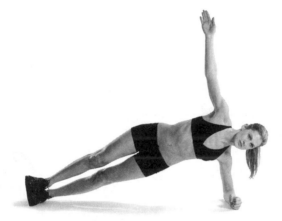

✳ Side Plank with Leg Raised

- Lift your right leg so your two legs form a V shape.
- Your torso should form a straight line from your neck through the midpoint of your pelvic floor.

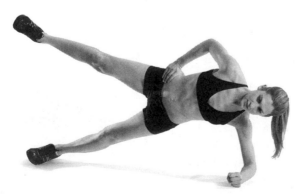

✳ Side Plank with Knee Tuck

- Lift your *left* leg, bend your left knee, and place the inside of your left foot beneath the inside of your right knee.
- Your body weight is now resting on your left forearm and the inside edge of your *right* foot.
- However hard it looks, it's actually harder to do.

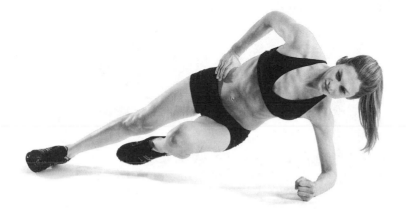

✳ Side Plank with Knee Tuck and Arm Overhead

- Combine the two variations for a side plank very few gym rats can hold for 30 to 45 seconds the first time they try it.

SIDE PLANK PROGRESSION SERIES #2: Feet elevated

✳ Side Plank with Feet Elevated

- Set up with your feet on a bench and your weight resting on your left forearm and the outside edge of your left foot.
- Your body should form a straight line from your neck through your ankles.

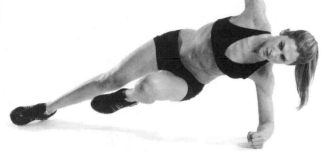

- If you're doing Phase One, Workout A, hold for 30 to 45 seconds.
- If you're doing Phase One, Workout B, hold for 10 seconds, relax for a second or two, and repeat.
- You can make this variation more challenging by lifting an arm overhead, raising your right leg, or both. Just make sure you double the padding under your left elbow. It's supporting almost all your body weight at this angle.
- Feeling masochistic? Try the side plank with knee tuck when your feet are elevated. Bend your left knee and hold your left foot under the inside of your right knee. Your weight rests on the inside edge of your right foot and your left forearm.

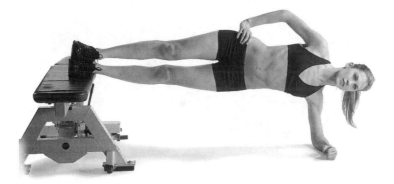

SIDE PLANK PROGRESSION SERIES #3: Feet elevated + unstable support

✳ Side Plank with Feet on Swiss Ball

- Set up with the outside of your left foot on the Swiss ball.
- If or when you can hold that position for 45 seconds (Workout A), or for 5 sets of 10-second holds on each side (Workout B), you can try any of the variations: right arm overhead, right leg raised, left knee tucked.

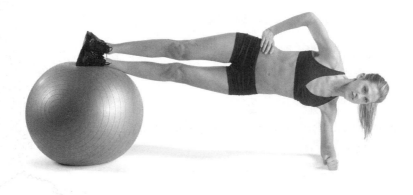

Alternative

✳ Side Plank with Feet Suspended

- Set up the TRX or equivalent so the ends are at least a few inches above the floor.
- Secure one or both feet in the straps. (I usually strap just one foot in, leaving the other one free for the masochistic variations.)
- Hold for 30 to 45 seconds if you're doing Workout A, or for 10-second sets if you're doing Workout B.

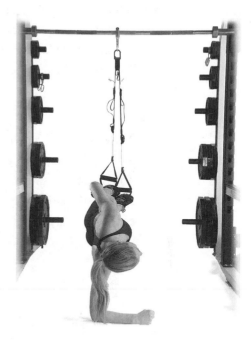

✳ Anti-Rotation Static Hold

GET READY

- I'm going to describe this as if everyone has access to a cable machine with an adjustable pulley. But you can do it just as easily with an exercise band, as long as you can attach it to something sturdy that's about 24 to 36 inches high.
- Attach a D-shaped handle to the cable, and set the pulley so it's about mid-thigh height.
- Grab the handle with both hands and kneel on both knees sideways to the cable machine. Straighten your torso so your body forms a straight line from your neck through your knees, and hold the handle with straight arms out in front of your chest.
- Keep your shoulders square.

HOLD

- Hold that position for 30 seconds.
- Relax, switch sides, and repeat.

THINK

- "Tall" and "tight." Keep your torso upright and eyes focused straight ahead.

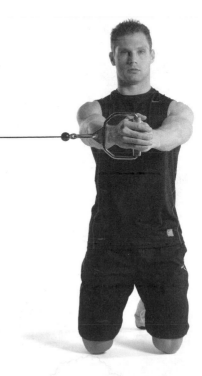

MODIFY

- To make the movement harder, add weight to the cable machine. If you're using a band, move farther away from whatever the band is attached to.
- To make it easier, reduce the weight, or move closer to the band's attachment point.

DON'T . . .

- Allow the shoulder closer to the machine to rise up. You have to keep your shoulders square to get all the benefits of the exercise. If you can't keep your shoulder down, you're using too much weight.
- Lean to the side, away from the resistance, to gain leverage. The point of the exercise is to stay upright against the resistance that's trying to pull you to that side.

Dynamic Stabilization

The goal of the stabilization chapter was to show you how to make progress—master one variation, then move up to the next. There's less emphasis on that in this chapter—only two of the seven exercises have sequences with increasing difficulty—mostly because the category itself is a progression.

Some of the exercises will be familiar and some will be new, but in all of them you're dealing with a new challenge: moving parts. The key to performing them successfully is to move the parts that are supposed to move, and *only* those parts. Simple enough, right? If only. You'll be cursing Alwyn, if not the entire fitness industry, before you're finished. You can't believe how challenging some of them are until you've given them your best shot.

When Alwyn first sent me the workouts, I told him I was unfamiliar with one of the dynamic-stabilization exercises. He steered me to a YouTube video that showed a trainer teaching it to one of his clients. The client couldn't do it without moving his entire torso, which defeats the purpose. But the trainer posted the video anyway. That means one of two things: Either the trainer didn't know how to do the exercise he was teaching (entirely possible, alas), or he couldn't find a client who could do it properly, and uploaded the attempt that came closest.

That doesn't mean *you* can't do it right. Alwyn wouldn't have put these moves in the workout if he didn't think you could master them. I'm just pointing out that some require patience and perseverance. Fortunately, the benefits you'll get—increased balance, coordination, and athleticism, in addition to the gains in core strength and endurance—more than make up for the learning curve.

✳ VALSLIDE PUSH-AWAY

GET READY

- You'll need a pair of Valslides—see page 61—and a carpeted floor. If you don't have Valslides, we'll show some variations you can try later in this chapter. I should note here that lots of things slide on carpet; I've done the push-away with my hands on Corelle dinner plates. If you're working out on a wood or tile floor, you can't use Valslides anyway (unless you also purchase booties for an extra $5), but towels might work almost as well.
- With a Valslide in each hand (the slick part goes on the carpet, in case that isn't obvious), get into a push-up position, with your weight resting on your hands and toes. Your arms are straight and your hands are about 2 inches in front of your shoulders.
- Your body should form a straight line from your neck through your ankles.

MOVE

- Slide your left arm straight ahead as far as you can without losing the neutral position of your lower back and pelvis.
- Pull it back, and slide out your right arm.
- Keep both arms straight throughout the movement.

THINK

- Focus on form, rather than range of motion. I can push a slide just 15 inches before I have to bend my elbows. (Yes, I got down on the floor and measured it.) That's with years of experience and practice doing this type of exercise. You might not get half that range of motion at first. Or you might get more; I'd never claim to represent the standard for excellence in anything. Just do the best you can without compromising your form.

DON'T . . .

- Rock your torso, as if you're trying to crawl, to extend your range of motion. You can move up to a more difficult variation once you feel you've maxed out on this one.

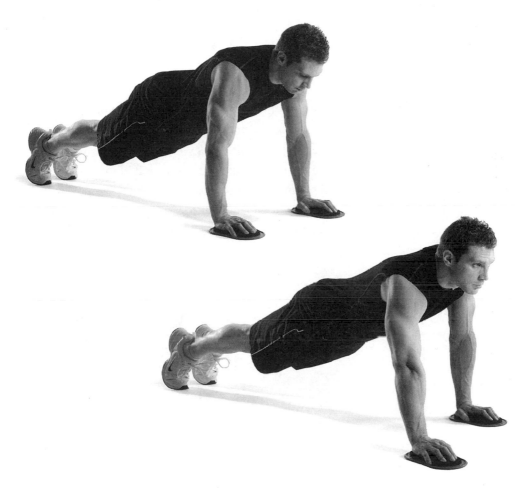

PUSH-AWAY PROGRESSION #1: Reduced base of support

✳ Push-Away with Leg Lift

- From the starting position, lift one leg so the toes are a few inches off the floor.
- Do half your repetitions, alternating arms on each rep, then switch legs and finish the set.

- You'll probably feel your torso pull to one side when you lift your dominant leg off the floor. Try to minimize the movement, but don't worry about eliminating it altogether. As long as your lumbar spine and pelvis remain in a neutral position, you're okay.

PUSH-AWAY PROGRESSION #2: Extended range of motion

✳ Push-Away with Bent Arms

- From the starting position, slide your left arm straight ahead as far as you can, bending your right elbow as your torso moves down toward the floor.
- Pull your left arm back to the starting position as you straighten your right arm.
- Slide your right arm out as far as you can, bending your left elbow.
- Return to the starting position, and finish the set.
- At the full range of motion, this variation is similar to a one-arm push-up, and thus requires a lot of upper-body strength. Be patient and do what you can when you can.

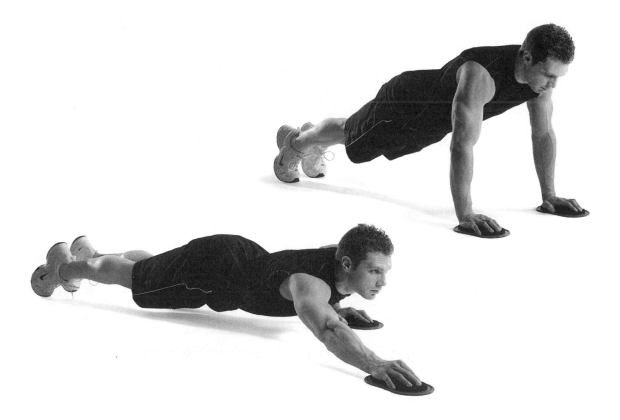

PUSH-AWAY PROGRESSION #3: Extended range of motion + reduced base of support

✳ Push-Away with Bent Arms + Leg Lift

- From the starting position, lift one leg so the toes are a few inches off the floor.
- Do half your repetitions, alternating arms on each rep, then switch legs and finish the set.
- This is an extremely challenging variation. As I write this, I'm still trying to get a full range of motion with one foot off the floor.
- There are other variations that are even more challenging than this one, but they're so difficult it's hard to imagine that any readers will need them to get the full benefits of this part of the program.

What Counts as a Rep?

When you do a unilateral exercise in a workout—a one-arm row or one-leg deadlift, for example—you expect to do the designated number of repetitions with each limb. If it's a set of 12, that means 12 with each arm or leg. Because you end up doing twice as many total repetitions, unilateral exercises are uniquely effective (which is to say uniquely exhausting) in fat-loss and conditioning programs.

But when you're doing the push-away variations shown here, you break that rule. Slide your left arm out, that's a rep. Slide your right arm out, that's another rep. If you're shooting for an even number, like 10 or 12, but hit the wall and have to stop on 9 or 11, note which arm did the last repetition, and start with the opposite one the next time you do the workout.

This only applies to push-away variations. For all the other dynamic-stabilization exercises that require equal work on both sides, you do the full number of reps with each arm or leg, or in each direction.

Alternative #1

✳ Walkout from Push-Up Position

If you don't have or want to purchase Valslides, you can do a similar exercise with no equipment at all.

- Start in the push-up position, with your hands about 2 inches in front of your shoulders.
- Walk your hands out as far as you can, then walk back to the starting position. That's one repetition.
- Continue until you finish the set.

✷ Walkout from Push-Up Position + Leg Lift

- From the push-up position, lift one leg, and then walk your hands out as far as you can. Continue as above.

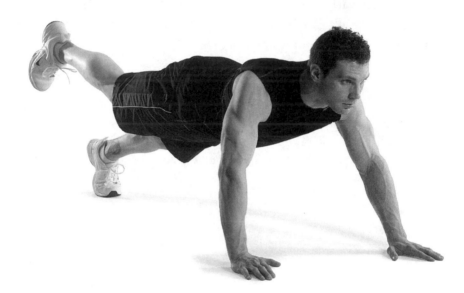

Alternative #2

✷ Swiss-Ball Rollout

- Set up as you would for the Swiss-ball plank, with your forearms on the ball and your weight resting on your forearms and toes. You probably want to start with your feet a comfortable distance apart.
- Unlike the plank, you won't start out with your body in a straight line from your neck through your ankles. Your hips will form a slight hinge, with your lumbar spine and pelvis in the neutral position.

- Roll the ball forward slowly and carefully, straightening your arms and going as far as you can while keeping your back and pelvis neutral.
- You may or may not straighten your hips as you do the exercise; it's completely individual. I'll just note that it's extremely difficult to get to the end range of motion, with your arms straight, without at least a slight amount of flexion in your hips.
- Pull the ball back to the starting position, and repeat.

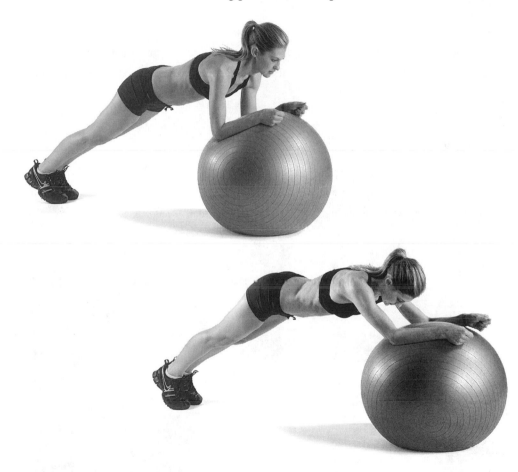

Alternative #2

✳ Suspended Fallout

- Attach a TRX or equivalent to a chin-up bar or something equally sturdy.
- Adjust the straps so the handles are about 36 inches above the floor.

- Grab the handles and position yourself so you're in push-up position, with your weight supported by your hands and toes and your hands about 2 inches in front of your shoulders.
- As with the Swiss-ball rollout, your hips will create a slight hinge in the starting position, with your lower back and pelvis set in the neutral position. You'll probably maintain that small amount of hip flexion throughout the exercise.
- Slowly and carefully fall forward, stopping when you feel you've gone as far as you can without losing your neutral spine position.
- Pull yourself back to the starting position, and repeat.
- You can make the exercise progressively harder first by extending your range of motion, and then by lowering the handles so they're closer to the floor. You can also lift one foot off the floor.

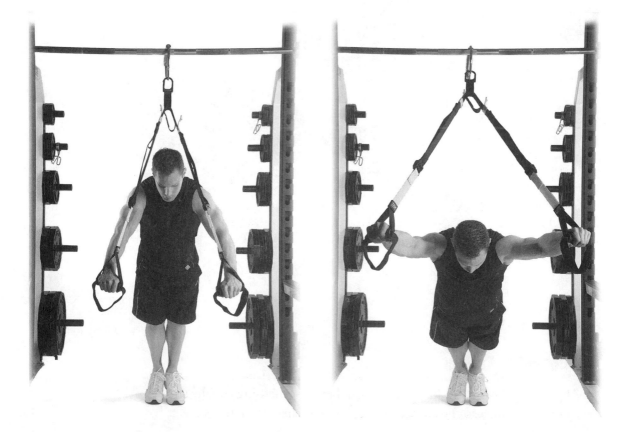

Some Rollouts Are More Equal than Others

The ab wheel, a lawn mower wheel with a plastic handle on each side, has a strange history among gym rats. Most of us knew what they were long before we ever considered using them. We'd walked past them countless times in sporting-goods stores. I don't know if it was the slick packaging, the $10 price tag, or the fact that we thought sit-ups and crunches were all we needed to work our abs, but whatever the reason, we just weren't into them.

But in 2000, in a book called *Bullet-proof Abs*, author and trainer Pavel Tsatsouline featured rollouts prominently. Within a few years you could find the wheels in health clubs, and today their efficacy as core-training devices is backed up by serious research, as I noted in Chapter 2. I've used the ab-wheel rollout off and on over the years.

The rollout is an anti-extension exercise, a category that includes the planks and push-aways that are key components of Alwyn's workouts. That is, you're training your core muscles to resist a sudden movement that forces your lumbar spine out of its neutral position and into hyperextension—an exaggerated arch.

So why isn't it in *NROL for Abs*? The problem is progression, or a lack of it. You can get really good at performing an exercise like the rollout from your knees, but how do you increase the challenge? I once tried to do a rollout from my feet, and ended up with my face flat on the floor. Only pure, dumb luck protected me from a concussion. (My ego, on the other hand, suffered multiple fractures.) At that moment, I learned there's no systematic way to advance from your knees to your feet on an anti-extension exercise. It's too big a jump to take with no steps in between.

Conversely, it's easy to make incremental progress with anti-rotation exercises, including the chops and lifts in this chapter and the static hold in Chapter 5. You can advance from kneeling to half-kneeling to standing, and you can adjust the weight incrementally as you get better at the exercises. You never have to increase the challenge in a dramatic way.

Alwyn's position is by no means universal. Lots of coaches and trainers use anti-extension exercises from the knees with their clients, and they're certainly popular in gyms these days. But if the goal is to make progressive improvement, it's better to use exercises on which you can progressively improve.

✳ Swiss-Ball Mountain Climber

GET READY

- Place your hands on a Swiss ball, roughly 18 to 24 inches apart.
- Set up as you would for a push-up hold, with your body forming a straight line from your neck to your ankles.

MOVE

- Raise your left foot off the floor and slowly bring your left knee up toward your chest.
- Lower it, and repeat with your right leg. That's one repetition.

THINK

- "One moving part." You want your torso and shoulders in the same position throughout the exercise. That's why you need to start with slow movements, allowing you to be aware of your posture, and notice any small deviation.
- Focus on hip flexion—using your hip-flexor muscles to pull your thigh up toward your chest.

DON'T . . .

- Rush through the exercise out of boredom. Yes, doing 10 to 12 slow repetitions of an exercise called "mountain climber" is a lot less exciting than climbing an actual mountain. But it's only one set, every other workout. The goal is to learn how to activate your hip flexors without compromising your spinal stability. The more you develop that ability, the better your back will perform in everything from running to team sports to, yes, actual mountain climbing.

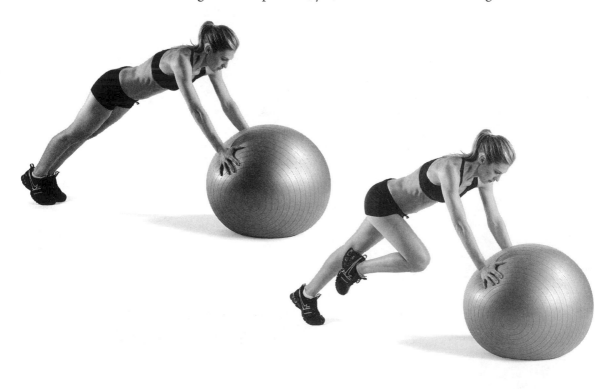

✳ ADVANCE

This is one of the more versatile exercises in the program. You can do it with your hands on the floor, on a bench, or on a medicine ball. You can do it with your feet on Valslides or a Swiss ball. You can do it with your arms or legs suspended—or maybe both, if you have the right equipment. And of course you can mix and match those variations any number of ways.

Those all would be interesting and challenging, but you aren't going to do them in this program. Instead, Alwyn wants you to adjust one variable: speed. When you're completely proficient at the slow-motion mountain climber (or simply bored out of your mind with it), start moving your legs faster. Just don't compromise your posture. That's unsafe at any speed.

✳ Cable Half-Kneeling Chop

GET READY

- Affix a rope handle to the high cable pulley. Slide the rope through its metal attachment ring as far as you can, giving you about 24 inches of rope to grasp.
- Grab the rope with an overhand grip, your hands as far apart as you can get them.
- Kneel sideways to the machine, with the knee closest to the machine up and the other one down. Your weight is resting on your inside foot and outside knee. (Make sure you have a mat beneath your knee, if you're working on a non-carpeted floor.)
- Straighten your torso to make yourself as tall as possible.
- Hold the rope between the machine and your shoulders.

MOVE

- Without rotating your torso, pull the rope slowly down and across your upper body. Your inside hand should end up in front of your outside hip.
- Return to the starting position, along the same diagonal line, again without rotating your torso.
- Do all your reps, switch sides, and repeat.

THINK

- "No rush." Make all your reps slow and deliberate, with complete focus on your form.

DON'T . . .

- Load up the exercise with a weight that forces you to twist your shoulders and crunch your abs to finish the set. Of course you can and should increase the weight you use as you improve, but never add weight at the expense of form. Your arms should be the only moving parts on this version of the exercise. There are other versions that become total-body movements, but that's not what you're doing in this phase of the program.

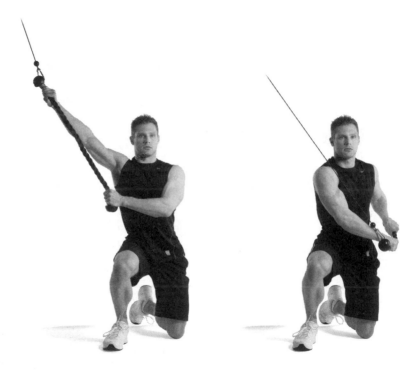

✳ Front Plank and Pulldown

GET READY

- Attach a D-shaped handle to the low cable pulley.
- Set up in a plank position facing the cable machine, with your weight resting on your forearms and toes, and your body forming a straight line from your neck to your ankles. You probably want to spread your feet so they're wider than your shoulders.
- Grab the handle with your right hand, using a neutral grip (your thumb on top, pinky on the bottom).

MOVE

- Without moving your torso, pull the handle until it's just below your right shoulder.
- Return to the starting position, again without moving your torso.
- Do all your reps, switch sides, and repeat.

THINK

- "Plank position."
- Your hips and shoulders must stay on a plane that's parallel to the floor, despite having just three points of support instead of four.

DON'T . . .

- Load up the machine with so much weight that you have to twist your shoulders and contract your abs to finish your reps. Use your ab muscles for stability only, and make your lat and arm muscles provide the movement.

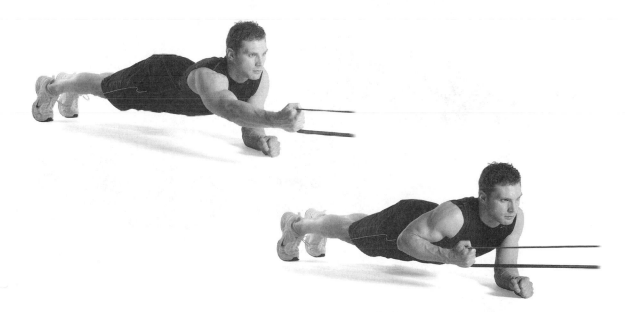

✳ Side Plank and Row

GET READY

- Attach a D-shaped handle to the low cable pulley.
- Set up in a side-plank position facing the cable machine, your weight resting on your left forearm and the outside edge of your left foot.
- Grab the handle with your right hand, your palm toward the floor.

MOVE

- Without moving your torso, pull the handle until it's at or near the right side of your rib cage.
- Return to the starting position, again without moving your torso.
- Do all your reps, switch sides, and repeat.

THINK

- Imagine that there's a wall behind your shoulders, preventing you from leaning back to finish each rep.

DON'T . . .

- Move at a speed that allows the weight to jerk you forward as you return to the starting position on each rep. Although the lats are doing the work, this isn't primarily a lat-building exercise. The goal is to make those muscles work while maintaining core stability.

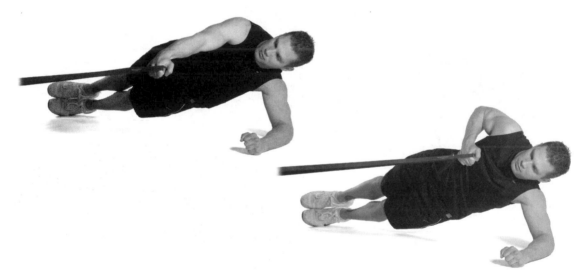

✳ Swiss-Ball Jackknife

GET READY

- Set up as you would for a Swiss-ball push-up hold, with your hands on the floor and your lower legs on the Swiss ball.
- You want your shins and the tops of your feet flat on the ball, with your knees off the ball and free to move.
- Your body should form a straight line from neck to ankles.

MOVE

- Without moving your torso, pull the ball forward so your thighs move toward your chest.
- Push the ball back to the starting position, again without moving your torso, and repeat.

THINK

- Picture a ceiling right above your hips, preventing you from lifting them.
- The technique here is different from what we showed in *NROL for Women*. In that one, the model raised her hips and contracted her abs, combining two movements: hip flexion and trunk flexion. Here we just want hip flexion, with your knees bending to allow the ball to roll forward.

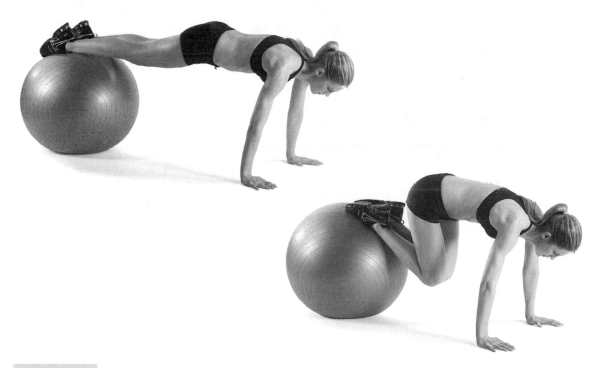

Alternative

✳ Swiss-Ball Pike

- Set up as you would for a Swiss-ball jackknife, with your shins and the tops of your feet flat on the ball.
- Keep your legs straight as you lift your hips toward the ceiling, pulling the ball

forward until your toes are on top of the ball. Your lower back and pelvis remain in the neutral position.

- Lower your hips as you return to the starting position, still keeping your legs straight.
- The pike is a lot harder than the jackknife, but it's not presented here as a progression. For some of you, the jackknife will be too easy, and you'll need to start with the pike. But for many others, perhaps most, the pike requires so much balance and coordination, in addition to the demands on core muscles, that it's not realistic to suggest readers try to master it during this phase of the program.

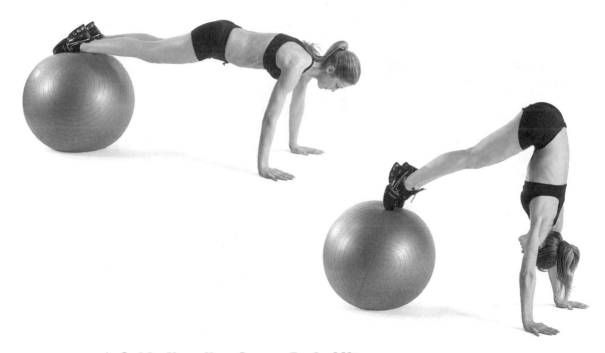

✳ Cable Kneeling Cross-Body Lift

GET READY

- Affix a rope handle to the low cable pulley. Slide the rope through its metal attachment ring as far as you can, giving you about 24 inches of rope to grasp.
- Grab the rope with an overhand grip, your hands as far apart as you can get them.
- Kneel sideways to the machine, holding the rope between the machine and the hip closest to the machine.
- Straighten your torso to make yourself as tall as possible.

MOVE

- Without rotating your torso, pull the rope slowly up and across your upper body. Your inside hand should end up just past your outside shoulder.
- Return to the starting position, along the same diagonal line, again without rotating your torso.
- Do all your reps, switch sides, and repeat.

THINK

- "No rush." As with the half-kneeling chop shown earlier, you want to make all your reps slow and deliberate, with complete focus on your form.

DON'T . . .

- Load up the exercise with a weight that forces you to twist your shoulders and crunch your abs to finish the set.

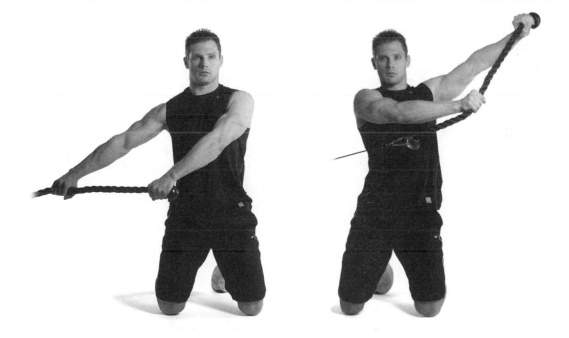

Integrated Stabilization

You won't see many options, progressions, or variations for the exercises in this category, for three reasons:

1. Each exercise is a progression from the ones you did in the dynamic stabilization category—in some cases, a *major* progression.
2. These exercises have a lot of moving parts. While some are based on movements you already know how to do—walking, for example—others are completely novel. The only thing in your life that could prepare you for the Turkish get-up is a history of doing Turkish get-ups. It's a great exercise, but if you've never done it before, you'll spend multiple workouts to reach the point at which it starts to feel natural.
3. You'll make progress by either adding weight or increasing speed. You don't need advanced versions of the exercises to get advanced results.

If you're feeling adventurous, the exercises in this category will turn your gym into an amusement park, albeit one in which you supply your own power for the best rides.

And if you're not feeling adventurous? Let me put it this way: Ever wonder why there's almost always a line for the machines that require no learning curve, little coordination, and hardly any effort if you don't feel like pushing the buttons that make it challenging? Conversely, you're much less likely to have to wait for the equipment that requires the most strength, skill, and effort.

These are the exercises that no one else is doing, in large part because very few people have ever seen them. I'm older than dirt and I've been working out since before the invention of mud, and I'd never done a couple of them before Alwyn included them in this program. But even after people see them, chances are you won't have a lot of imitators in your local health club. Fact is, they tend to create *just a bit* of social distance. They don't look like the exercises everyone else is doing.

On the bright side, social distance often translates into physical distance. People give you space when you move in ways they haven't seen before. So you get two major benefits from integrated-stabilization exercises:

First, you get the considerable benefits of the exercises, including improved balance, coordination, conditioning, and athleticism in addition to the obvious core strength and endurance. Second, people get the hell out of your way when you do never-before-seen exercises like alligator drags and farmer's walks while holding mismatched dumbbells over your head.

✳ Turkish Get-Up

GET READY

- You'll need a dumbbell or, even better, a kettlebell.
- Lie flat on your back on the floor, holding the weight in your left hand straight over your chest, with your left elbow locked. Your palm is turned toward your toes. If you're using a kettlebell, the round base rests on the part of your forearm that's closest to your face.
- Your left knee is bent, with your left foot up near your butt and your toes turned out slightly. Your right arm is out at a 45-degree angle, with your right palm flat on the floor. Your right leg is straight.
- Your eyes are on the weight, where they'll stay for the entire movement. Stare at that thing like it's a naked movie star.

FIRST MOVE

- Push down hard with your left heel, pushing your body to the right as you bend your right arm and support your weight on your right elbow and forearm. This part is literally like getting up out of bed, except for the fact that you're holding a weight.
- Now rise from your right elbow to your right hand, which you slide behind you at a 45-degree angle.

SECOND MOVE

- Push down with your left heel and right hand, lifting your torso and hips off the floor.
- Bring your right leg up under your body, and then rest your right knee on the floor, so you're now in a half-kneeling position, with your left knee forward and your left foot still flat on the floor.

THIRD MOVE

- Stand up.

FINISH

- Reverse your movements to return to the starting position.
- Finish your reps with your left arm holding the weight, then repeat with your right arm.

DON'T . . .

- Obsess over achieving perfect form. If the arm holding the weight stays overhead, and you manage to get up to your feet and then back down to the floor again, that's close enough. It's okay to let your muscles figure out the details on their own. In a way, that's the point of integrated stabilization. You've trained your core muscles to support your spine, and now you have to set them loose.
- Worry about using heavy weights—not at first, anyway. You can find Internet pictures and videos of athletes doing TGUs with loaded barbells, but you don't have to match their feats to get the benefits of the exercise. I especially recommend using a light dumbbell or kettlebell the first time you try it. If you're able to get up and down smoothly and easily while keeping your working arm locked and perpendicular to the floor, go ahead and challenge yourself with heavier weights.

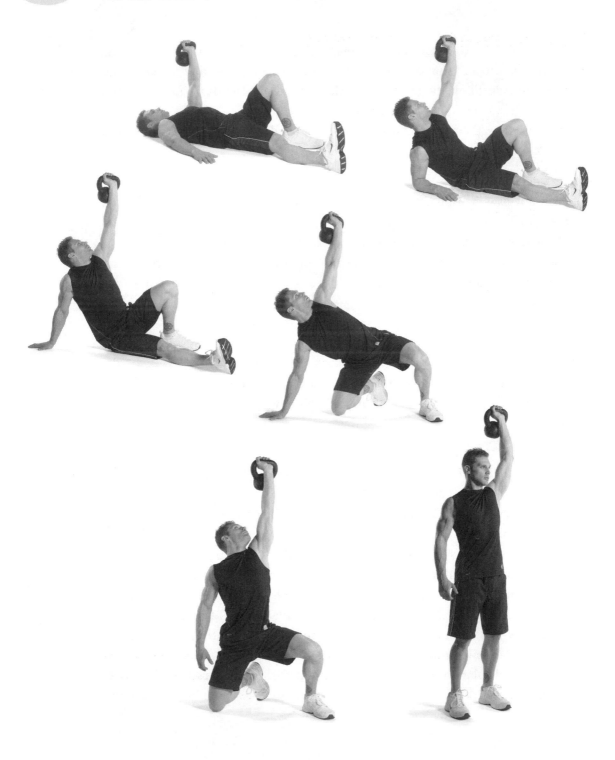

✳ Suitcase Deadlift + Lateral Step-Up

GET READY

- You'll need a dumbbell and a sturdy box to step up on. The box can be any height, depending on how challenging you want the exercise to be. I suggest using a six-inch box the first time, and then going up from there when you're familiar with the exercise.
- Stand with the box just outside your left foot, holding the dumbbell in your right hand at arm's length to your side. Your feet are about hip-width apart, with your toes pointed forward.

MOVE

- Squat down until the weight is a few inches from the floor, keeping your back and pelvis in the neutral position and your shoulders square.
- As you stand back up, take a wide step to the left and plant your left foot on the box, followed by your right. Stand up straight, with your feet hip-width apart.
- Take a wide step to the right to return to the starting position.
- Finish all the reps with the weight in your right hand, then repeat the set, holding the weight in your left hand and stepping up on the box to your right.

THINK

- Regard this as one fluid movement. The deadlift and lateral step-up flow directly into the lateral step-down and the next repetition of the deadlift. When you first try it, you'll probably come to a very brief pause when both feet are on the step, and then pause again when both feet are back on the floor. But in subsequent workouts, make all your reps on one side a continuous movement, and then after you switch sides, make those reps another nonstop movement.

DON'T . . .

- Allow your body to tilt to either side as you do the exercise. Don't lean to the left when doing a suitcase deadlift with the weight in your left hand, and don't bend to the right as you're stepping up. The core-training benefits come from having the unbalanced load to one side, followed by a step in the opposite direction.

● Make it too easy on yourself. A light weight is fine the first time you try it, but once you know how to do the exercise, you won't get much out of it if the weight isn't challenging your balance and stability. You can also make it more difficult by using a higher step. But if you go with a light weight and low step throughout the program, you may as well be doing step aerobics.

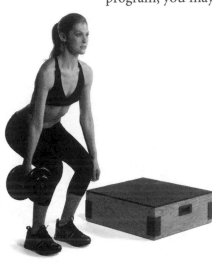

✴ Cable Anti-Rotation Reverse Lunge with Chop

GET READY

- Attach a D-shaped handle to the high cable pulley.
- Stand with your right side toward the machine, holding the handle above and outside your right shoulder.
- Your feet are about hip-width apart, toes pointed forward.
- Your eyes should stay focused straight ahead throughout the movement.

MOVE

- Step back with your left leg into a lunge position.
- At the same time, pull the cable down and across your torso in a diagonal pattern, while keeping your shoulders and hips square.
- As you stand back up, return the cable to the starting position, reversing the diagonal pattern.
- Finish all the reps, switch sides, and repeat.

DON'T . . .

- Twist your shoulders and crunch your abs to finish the chop. You have to use a weight that's light enough to allow your torso to stay upright and your shoulders to remain square.

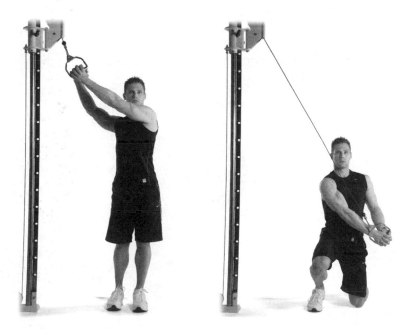

✳ Alligator Drag

GET READY

- Grab a pair of Valslides, and find a stretch of carpeted floor that allows you to go forward 10 to 20 yards. If you don't have Valslides, you can use anything that will slide over the surface with minimal drag or friction. Dinner plates or plastic bags might work on a carpeted floor, while towels might work on wood or tile.
- Get into push-up position with your feet on the slides.

MOVE

- Walk yourself forward with your hands to the end of your runway.
- If you've gone at least 10 yards, or as far as you can before pooping out, consider that one set. Rest, then repeat the alligator walk back to where you started.
- If you can't go 10 yards in one direction, go as far as you can, then immediately switch positions and return to the starting point without resting. You want to go at least 10 yards for each set.

THINK

- Your legs and feet are just along for the ride. No, it's not exactly how an alligator moves (I know you herpetologists are sticklers for that sort of thing), but it's still fun to try, and fun to see the looks on the faces of your fellow lifters the first time you drag yourself around the gym.

DON'T . . .

- Allow your hips to sag and your lower back and pelvis to drop out of the neutral position.

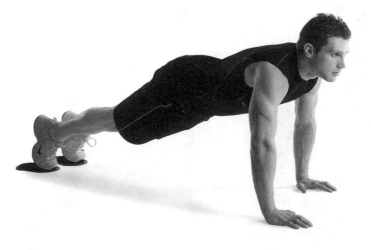

✳ Dumbbell Offset Farmer's Walk

GET READY

- Grab a single, relatively heavy dumbbell, and stand someplace where you can walk 10 to 20 steps.
- Hold the dumbbell either at your side (as you did for the suitcase deadlift) or at your shoulder. Either way, hold it with your palm turned toward your body.

MOVE

- Walk forward to the end of your path.
- If you've gone at least 10 steps, or as far as you can before fatiguing, consider that one set. Rest, switch the weight to the other side, then repeat the farmer's walk back to where you started.
- If you can't go 10 steps in one direction, go as far as you can, then immediately turn around and return to the starting point without resting. You want to go at least 10 steps for each set.

DON'T . . .

- Lean toward the side holding the weight, or lean the opposite direction to improve your leverage. You want an upright posture, with your shoulder and hips square and facing the direction of your walk.

Alternative #1

✳ Dumbbell Offset Squat

- If you don't have a clear path to walk, you can do squats instead, holding the weight at your side or at your shoulder.
- Do 10 to 20 squats while holding the weight on each side, taking a short rest in between.

Alternative #2

✳ Two-Dumbbell Offloaded Farmer's Walk or Squat

- You can do either of these exercises holding two dumbbells of unequal weight, either at your sides or at your shoulders.

- After 10 to 20 steps or reps, switch the weights, and do the same number of steps or reps with the heavier weight on the opposite side.

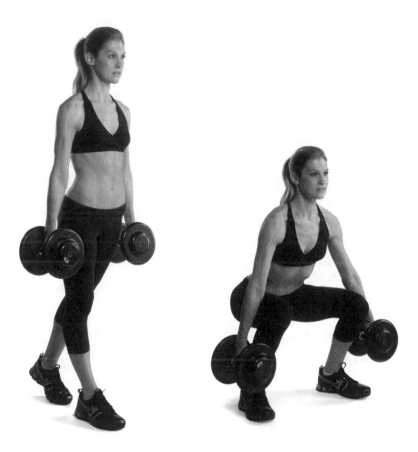

✳ Dumbbell Overhead Offloaded Farmer's Walk or Squat

GET READY

- Grab two dumbbells, one about 10 pounds heavier than the other, and hold them overhead, with your palms facing each other.

MOVE

- Walk forward 10 to 20 steps, or do 10 to 20 squats.
- Rest, then switch the weights and repeat the set.

DON'T...

- Get upset when half the people in the weight room ask if you know you're using mismatched dumbbells. Smile, tell them you're doing it on purpose as part of your core training, and get on with your workout. If they won't accept the truth, it's your moral obligation to make up something interesting. ("It's my religion—we face Los Angeles and feel the burn.")

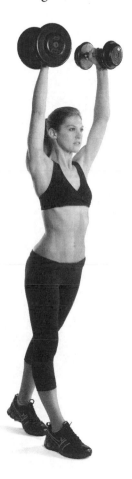

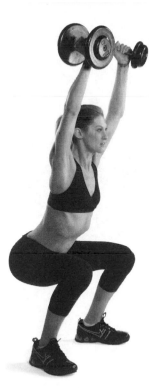

PART 3

ALL TRAINING IS CORE TRAINING

8

Strength,
in Numbers

ALWYN'S WORKOUTS in *NROL for Abs* have four components:

1. DYNAMIC WARM-UP

You have two primary goals:

(a) Warm up your body in the literal sense—increase your core temperature, speed up your heart rate, and dilate your blood vessels so they can more efficiently move nutrients and metabolites in and out of your muscles.

(b) Prepare your joints for the upcoming workout by moving them through their full range of motion.

You may also accomplish two secondary goals: Your overall conditioning and athleticism probably will improve, especially if you aren't used to the exercises. And you'll either maintain or improve your mobility. Since that's the subject of Chapter 9, I'll leave it there for now.

This part of the workout takes about 10 minutes.

2. CORE TRAINING

You know from reading chapters 4, 5, 6, and 7 that Alwyn's program includes three levels of core training, which you'll do sequentially: stabilization, dynamic stabilization, and integrated stabilization. This should also take about 10 minutes.

3. STRENGTH TRAINING

The strength program, the subject of this chapter, also has three levels. Because I've exceeded my jargon allowance, these levels are called Phase One, Phase Two, and Phase Three. Core and strength training are synched up by design, so you'll do stabilization exercises in Phase One, dynamic stabilization in Phase Two, and integrated stabilization in Phase Three. The strength workout should last about 20 minutes.

3A. POWER TRAINING

In Phase Three, Alwyn includes this bonus exercise category, which consists of one or two exercises per workout, and which you'll do in between core and strength training. "Power" and "strength" are often used interchangeably, but technically they mean different things. *Strength* is the ability to move a weight, regardless of the speed at which it moves. *Power* is the ability to move a weight fast. The two are related, but from time to time it's good to train them in isolation.

Everyone should do at least the first power exercise in each workout of Phase Three. The second exercise involves throwing a medicine ball to the floor or against a wall, which most of us can't do at home or in a commercial gym. Do that exercise if you can, but don't worry if you can't.

4. METABOLIC TRAINING

In years past, this category would've been labeled "cardio," "fat loss," or "energy-systems work." Alwyn prefers "metabolic training" because the goal is to push the limits of your metabolism, to make your body work harder, with the goal of burning off more of its stored energy, which it will have to replace later in the day as you recover. This keeps your metabolism elevated—you're burning more calories post-workout than if you'd done easier, steady-paced exercise—and makes your body use a higher percentage of fat calories during that recovery.

As you probably guessed, metabolic training only works if it's difficult. You have to take something out of your body before your metabolism will kick into a higher gear to replace it. No drain, no gain.

I'm not saying your workouts have to be debilitating. But you do have to leave your comfort zone during this portion of the workout. You have to breathe hard and feel the prickles of thousands of your sweat glands opening to keep your body from overheating.

You won't start metabolic training until Phase Two of the program. There's a learning curve in Phase One that requires more time and energy than you'd expect. You're doing new exercises, and doing them in a new way. You're also developing a base of core strength and endurance, which you'll need before you start pushing your body this hard.

Metabolic work will take between 10 and 20 minutes to complete.

HOW IT WORKS

The NROL for Abs program, as you know, has three phases. Each phase includes two separate workouts. These are labeled Workout A and Workout B. You'll alternate between these workouts until you finish the phase. Under no circumstances will you do both workouts on the same day, or even on consecutive days. You need at least one full day off after each workout.

For best results, you want to do Alwyn's workouts two or three times a week. Since these are total-body workouts—working all your major muscles each time you go to the gym—you won't be able to recover effectively from one session to the next if you train more than three times a week. And fewer than two weekly workouts just isn't enough training to get the results you want.

If you typically work out on Monday, Wednesday, and Friday, your training schedule would look like this:

	Monday	Tuesday	Wednesday	Thursday	Friday	Saturday	Sunday
Week 1	Workout A	off	Workout B	off	Workout A	off	off
Week 2	Workout B	off	Workout A	off	Workout B	off	off
Week 3	Workout A	off	Workout B	off	Workout A	off	off
Week 4	Workout B	off	Workout A	off	Workout B	off	off

Or you could do the workouts on Tuesday, Thursday, and Saturday. Whatever works.

You want to do each workout in each phase at least six times. If you're relatively inexperienced in the weight room, or if you just really like one of the phases, you can do each of the workouts as many as eight times. It's your choice.

That means each phase will take four to eight weeks to complete. If you have to

What to Do on "Off" Days

Of the twenty-eight days shown in the chart, just twelve are designated for workouts. The other sixteen are labeled "off" days. I strongly encourage you to get some type of physical activity on those days. Walk around the neighborhood with your dog, take a bike ride with your kids, or go off for a solo run. Prefer to do something athletic? Hit some tennis balls with your spouse, shoot some hoops in the driveway, spend some time in the batting cage, or hit a bucket of balls at the driving range.

Some activities offer more benefits than others, as I show in Chapter 17, and with benefits come risks. But that's really beside the point. Doing *something* is the key. As long as you shut off your computer, turn off the TV, set aside the cell phone, and get up and move, you're on the right track. (You'll learn why in Chapter 13.) You can move fast or slow. You can do something purposeful or random. It can be competitive or cooperative or solitary. It absolutely, totally *does not matter*. Just do something that involves physical movement and that gets you away from work and electronic entertainment.

And don't just do this on your "off" days. It's best to do it every single day, even the days when you hit the gym.

stop for a week or two due to illness or unexpected events, just pick up where you left off.

HOW TO DO THE WORKOUTS

If you've done the workouts in either or both of the previous *NROL* books, you can skim through this section. For everyone else, the charts, directives, and nomenclature can be a bit intimidating at first. Let's walk through each component.

Workouts

A workout is what you do in one session. In *NROL for Abs*, it includes all the elements I mentioned at the start of this chapter: dynamic warm-up, core, strength, power (in Phase Three), and metabolic training (in Phase Two and Phase Three).

Exercises

Exercises are usually listed as pairs. In the workout charts in Chapter 10, you'll see that the strength exercise pairs are designated 1a and 1b or 2a and 2b. Here's an example from Phase One, Workout A:

Exercise	Sets	Reps	Rest (seconds)
1a: Split squat, front foot elevated	2–3	12 (each leg)	45–60
1b: Inverted row	2–3	12	45–60
2a: Romanian deadlift	2–3	12	45–60
2b: Push-up	2–3	12	45–60

You might have heard the word "superset" used to describe pairs of exercises, and that's accurate as far as it goes. But when most people think of supersets, they think of two or more exercises performed back to back without rest in between. That's not what you're doing here. Alwyn prefers to call them "alternating sets," or "alternating sets with full rest." You do the first exercise in a pair (1a or 2a), rest for the time suggested in the workout chart, then do the next exercise (1b or 2b). Rest again, then go back to 1a or 2a and repeat.

If an exercise just has a number, with no letter following it, that means you do "straight sets." That is, you do all of the designated work for that exercise, resting for the appropriate amount of time between sets, then move on to the next exercise.

One question that always comes up is what to do when you don't have the equipment necessary for an exercise. I've tried to include alternatives to everything that calls for equipment you may not have at home, or that some gyms may not have readily available. At a minimum, whether you work out at home or a gym, you should have access to:

- barbell with weight plates
- dumbbells (adjustable or fixed)
- chin-up bar or equivalent
- cable system or elastic band(s)
- bench
- step or box that's lower than a bench
- Swiss ball
- some kind of clock, watch, or timer

If you work out at home and don't have a cable system, I highly recommend buying at least one exercise band. Some of the most important exercises require one or the other, and there really aren't any alternative ways to replicate the type of resistance that cables and bands provide. I promise you this up front: Neither Alwyn nor I will answer any question from a reader that starts with, "I work out at home and don't have bands or a cable machine . . ." You just have to skip those exercises if you can't or won't acquire the equipment you need.

Sets, Reps, and Rest

A repetition, or rep, is a single execution of an exercise—one push-up or chin-up or lunge or squat. A set is a collection of reps. Alwyn's workouts usually specify how many sets and reps to do for each exercise, although there are exceptions. Some of the core exercises describe an amount of time to hold a position. In those cases, a set is completed when you've held the position for at least the minimum amount of time.

You'll also see a suggested amount of time to rest between sets—30 to 45 seconds, for example. Readers inevitably ask if they have to rest that exact amount of time. Honestly, you don't *have* to do anything. Alwyn uses specific numbers because, in his experience and judgment (keep in mind that he has a lot of the former and is highly regarded for the latter), this is the time it typically takes for a lifter to recover well enough to do the next set with the intensity required to get all the benefits of the program.

Of course you can decide for yourself if those rest periods are right for you. Some, like me, prefer short rest periods because we're impatient and like to keep moving. Others might take more time because they're using heavier weights and achieving a deeper level of fatigue on each set. No matter how hard we try to comply with the guidelines, at some point we all gravitate toward the way we prefer to train.

So why does Alwyn suggest a one-size-fits-all rest period? There are two types of lifters who will benefit.

If you're like me, and you typically go from one exercise to the next without much time in between, the success of your workout depends on cumulative fatigue. Whatever you sacrifice by not resting long enough to be near full strength on each set, you hope to make up with the metabolic disruption of forcing your muscles to work with incomplete recovery. It's a better formula for fat loss and muscle maintenance than for building size and strength, but it certainly works . . . as long as you're selecting your own exercises and choosing your own system of sets and reps.

Short-rest-period lifters get blindsided by Alwyn's workouts. His routines look simple enough on paper, but when you actually do his exercises in the order he arranges them, you realize you're accumulating more fatigue, and accumulating it faster, than you expected. So by not resting enough between sets of the first exercises in the workout, you have less energy for the last ones. This is true even when the entire strength workout is just four exercises. How you do the first two determines what you have left for the others.

Then there's the lifter who thinks every workout is "too easy." I'll give you an example: After *NROL for Women* came out in hardcover in 2008, I began getting bewildering e-mails from readers who didn't understand the programs and did multiple training sessions in a single workout. One of them, I kid you not, had done the equivalent of eight workouts. Her only complaint? The workouts took too long!

There's no way in the world readers like her were training with the level of intensity Alwyn had in mind when he created this program. (The readers who mistakenly did double workouts and trained with the required intensity told me they were devastated afterward—drained and sore to a degree that's highly counterproductive, and that Alwyn would never inflict on a client.) A single workout may not look like much on paper, but it should be a challenge to execute. Rest periods are one way to test your assumptions about how hard you're working. For example, in Phase One you're doing two or three sets of 12 reps of each exercise, with 45 to 60 seconds of rest in between. If you can't understand why anyone would need to rest more than 15 seconds, that's a sign *you didn't do the exercise right.* You need to increase the weight, or work at a less comfortable pace (slower or faster, depending on the exercise), or improve your form.

Weight

We don't tell you how much weight to use on the exercises that require an external load. If you're a relatively inexperienced lifter, you'll have to use trial and error to find the right weight. Even dedicated gym rats might over- or underestimate the amount they need. I don't think a single reader will have experience with every exercise in the program, so all of us have to use our best guesses.

My advice to experienced lifters:

Guys should deduct ten pounds from whatever they think their starting weight should be. If that's too light, go up ten pounds for the second set. Still too light? Add ten more pounds for the third set.

Women should add five to ten pounds to their first-set weight. If it's too heavy . . . oh, who am I kidding? It won't be too heavy; it might still be too light.

A weight is exactly right if you can do all the reps. On the first set, you want to feel as if you could've done two or three more. The second set should end with the feeling that *maybe* you could do one more. If the third set is your last one for that exercise, you shouldn't even get that final rep without a herculean effort. If you get all the reps on all your sets, and get them somewhat easily, it's a sign you're working with weights that are too light.

CHARTING YOUR WORKOUTS

You absolutely must keep a workout log. You can't make progress unless you know what you've already done. Progress usually means one of three things:

More reps. Let's say that on Monday, January 4, you do two sets of lat pulldowns with 85 pounds, and complete a total of 21 reps: 12 in the first set, 9 in the second. (Yes, you were pretty aggressive with your choice of a starting weight.) On Friday, January 8, you do 24 reps with that same weight: 12 in the first set, 12 in the second. Adding three reps from one workout to the next is a nice improvement.

More sets. On Wednesday, January 13, you add a set to each exercise, using the same weight. You get a total of 33 reps—12 in the first set, 12 in the second, 9 in the third. Thanks to that additional set, you improved by 9 reps.

More weight. On Monday, January 18, you do your lat pulldowns with 90 pounds instead of 85. You get 12 reps in the first set, 11 in the second, and 10 in the third. Those 33 reps equal your January 13 total, but because you used more weight, you've made progress.

There are two other ways to make progress within this program. One you already know: With the core exercises, you can do a more difficult or challenging variation of the exercise. The final system of progression comes into play in Phase Three. In those workouts, your goal is to do more sets and reps *within a specified block of time* from one workout to the next. (I'll explain the details when we get there, in Chapter 12.)

So that's why you keep a workout log. Now let's look at how you keep one.

THE NEW RULES OF LIFTING FOR ABS

Don't panic if you don't yet know what these exercises are. They're illustrated and explained in full detail in Chapter 10. All you need to focus on here is the process of keeping a training log. You can find blank training-log pages at NROLbooks.com, and if you can't remember that URL, just go to my website, louschuler.com, and I'll get you linked up. Or you can go to the official discussion forum for *NROL for Abs* at forums.jpfitness.com, and find your way from there.

Once you've downloaded and printed a set of blank log pages (you'll need sepa-

Phase: One Workout: A									
Exercise	Sets	Reps or time	Set #						Rest
			1	2	3	4	5	6	
Core training: stabilization									
1a: plank	2	60–90s	90s	75s					45–60 s
1b: side plank	2	30–45s	40s	30s					45–60 s
Strength									
1a: split squat, front foot elevated (DB)	2–3	12	20/12	20/11	20/8				45–60 s
1b: inverted row (Smith machine)	2–3	12	12	8	5				45–60 s
2a: Romanian deadlift (barbell)	2–3	12	95/12	95/12	95/10				45–60 s
2b: push-up (Smith machine)	2–3	12	12	12	12				45–60 s
Notes:									

rate pages for workouts A and B), the first thing you do is write down the exercises, plus the suggested sets and reps. That tells you what you *want* to do. As you work out, you'll record what you *actually* do.

In this workout, you started out doing basic planks and side planks. (This is after the dynamic warm-up, of course. You don't need to record the warm-up exercises on your training log.) The goal on the plank was to hold a static position for 60 to 90 seconds on each of two sets. You held for 90 seconds on the first set and 75 on the second, which is outstanding. Next time you do workout A, you should move up to a more advanced variation of the exercise.

Let's skip ahead to the exercise called "split squat, front foot elevated (DB)." If you don't already know, you'll learn what a split squat is in Chapter 10. (It's a stationary lunge, if that helps.) "Front foot elevated" means your front foot is on a box, rather than flat on the floor. "(DB)" means you're doing the exercise with dumbbells. Feel free to create and use your own abbreviations if you don't like mine.

The workout calls for two or three sets of 12 reps. You chose to do three. "20/12" means you used 20-pound dumbbells, and got 12 reps on the first set. For the second set, "20/11" shows you got 11 reps. Clearly, the weight was neither too light nor too heavy. You only got 8 reps on the third set ("20/8"), but that's not a problem. Fatigue hits us harder than we expect on some exercises, and this is certainly one of them.

Now let's look at the next exercise. "Inverted row" means you're face-up, pulling your body upward, rather than pulling something toward your body. "(Smith machine)" means you did the exercise on that device, which is a barbell that moves up and down on a fixed path. In this case, you would fix the barbell in one position, and use it as a pull-up bar in which your body is more horizontal than vertical.

You'll notice there's no designation for weight. That's because you're using your body weight only. When you need to make the exercise more or less difficult, you change the height of the bar. The lower it is, the harder it is to pull yourself up to it. You can make it even harder by raising one foot off the floor, or by elevating both feet onto a bench. That's not necessary in this case, because you managed just 12, 8, and 5 reps on your three sets. The next time you do this workout, you want to set the bar of the machine at the same height, and work to get more reps. Your goal is to get 12 reps on each set, then lower the bar to make it more challenging.

9

The Nobility of Mobility

LET'S REVISIT THE SCENARIO at the start of Chapter 1: "Your gym, six p.m. Monday. You find an unoccupied strip of carpet in the area reserved for warming up and doing ab exercises. The guy to your right . . ."

Stop the tape.

Instead of looking at the people around you doing crunches and planks, focus on the ones who're warming up. What do you see?

If you guessed "trick question," you're right. The ones doing crunches and planks *are* warming up. As is the young woman doing hamstring stretches on the floor, the older gentleman leaning against a wall to loosen up his calves, and maybe half the people on treadmills, stationary bikes, and elliptical machines. That's not to mention the men and women waiting in line to use those machines.

Everybody in this scenario knows you need to do *something* to prepare your body for a serious workout. Most of them understand that it should involve movement, which gets blood to muscles, increases heart rate, and elevates the body's core temperature. All of those processes are important. But no one seems interested in taking the next step: performing a warm-up routine that involves movement in multiple directions, works your joints through a range of motion, and stimulates your nervous system.

There are two good reasons why so few people go mobile:

First, health clubs aren't set up for it. The warm-up areas are designed for users to claim tiny strips of floor space for linear, stationary exercises like crunches and hamstring stretches. If you need to move, hey, that's what the treadmills are for. It's no coincidence that cardio machines use symmetrical rectangles of real estate that mirror the self-selected spaces in the warm-up areas. Really, what is a crowded health club but a configuration of implied rectangles to accommodate the simplest, most predictable, and most linear exercises? Try doing an exercise—any exercise—that re-quires a non-rectangular space and involves movements in multiple directions, and see how many dirty looks you get for disturbing the quadrilateral feng shui.

Second, people aren't set up for it. Nobody wants to be the rolling stone in a field of rectangular moss. (Well, some people do, but we have medications for them.) We only celebrate nonconformists in retrospect. In real time, we like people to do what we're doing, which more often than not is what everyone else is doing.

That's exactly why you need to be the one moving against the tide. You need to do exercises that are different from the ones other people are doing—not because they're different, but because they're *better*.

You and your fellow gym members have defaulted to a mediocre training para-digm because it's convenient and makes efficient use of the space. Who benefits from the convenience and efficiency? The people who own the gym. Who loses? You, me, and everyone else whose workout is based more on geometry than physiology.

Here's something Alwyn told me while we were working on this book: "If what readers were doing in a commercial gym worked, I'd be out of business, and we wouldn't need any books." He was even more to the point when we discussed the fact that the exercises in this chapter look different from what everyone else is doing to warm up: "I'm not going to write a program that I wouldn't give to someone who actually hired me. I'd be lying. It's just not authentic."

All that said, Alwyn's dynamic warm-up routine isn't as strange as my argument for it suggests. You'll see that most of the exercises involve the body's biggest muscles, literally warming them up with movement. They also do something else that's so important it needs its own rule.

NEW RULE #9 • Stability in your lower back depends on mobility in the joints above and below it.

In *Advances in Functional Training*, Mike Boyle describes the mobility-stability continuum. Starting with the ankles, "the joints alternate between mobility and stability," Boyle writes. Ankles need mobility, while knees need stability. If you follow sports, you know what happens when knees bend backward into hyperextension, or rotate. Either of those can be a ticket to the DL for an athlete, if not into retirement.

Then you have the hips, which require mobility, followed by the lumbar spine, which absolutely must acquire and maintain a very high degree of stability, as I've noted maybe a thousand times so far. But let's return to the hips: If your thigh bones can't move the way they're supposed to, with a long range of motion forward and backward and a somewhat shorter range to the side, then something else has to move instead. It might be your knees, your lumbar spine, or both.

That's why a complete core-training program starts with mobility exercises, which focus primarily on the hip joints. Only when you've warmed up and achieved the proper range of motion in your hips do you move on to stability exercises for the lower back.

But the hips aren't the only joints that can enhance or compromise core stability. You also need mobility in your thoracic spine, the joints just to the north of your lower back. Unlike the thick vertebrae of your lumbar spine, these joints need to rotate. If they didn't, you wouldn't be able to turn your shoulders without twisting your lumbar vertebrae, and that would either cause an injury or set you up for one.

Alwyn's warm-up routine starts with an exercise for your thoracic spine, followed by an exercise for your hips. If you could only do two warm-up exercises, these probably would qualify as the most important in the routine. But we hope you'll do more than two.

If you feel weird being the only person in the gym who's actually going from one place to another during your warm-up drills, you have two choices:

First, and best, is to find an unused group-exercise room, and move around as much as you need to. If anyone else is using the room during its downtime between classes, chances are good he or she is also doing exercises that don't fit neatly into the geometry of the warm-up area.

But let's say you work out at peak hours, when there's a full slate of yoga, Pilates, Zumba, Spinning, and whatever other classes might be popular as you read this. The gym is too crowded for you to carve your own path between the rectangles. That brings me to the second-best choice: Do stationary versions of the exercises within a traditional plot of warm-up turf. Instead of going ten yards to the left and ten yards to the right, alternate reps to the left and right without leaving your spot.

Some of the exercises, like the jumps and hops, will still look different from the things other people are doing. But that brings me back to my original point in this chapter: As Alwyn says, the "normal" stuff doesn't work well enough for most people to get the results they seek. *NROL for Abs* exists for one reason above all others: There's a better way to train. It starts with a dynamic warm-up.

Dynamic Warm-up • Use with A and B workouts.	
Exercise	**Reps/distance**
Bent-over thoracic extension and rotation	10 each direction
Squat to stand	5
Forward/backward jump	10 each direction
Crossover walking toe touch	10–20 yards
Lateral jump	10 each direction
Lateral cross-behind lunge	10–20 yards each direction
Seal jack	10
Reverse inchworm	5
Forward-backward hop	10 each direction, each leg
Curtsy lunge	10 each direction
Movement skills	
Straight-leg run	10–20 yards, repeated once
Side shuffle with arm cross	10–20 yards each direction
Butt kick	10–20 yards, repeated once

WARM-UP EXERCISES

✳ Bent-Over Thoracic Extension and Rotation

- Stand with your feet shoulder-width apart and arms out to your sides.
- Bend forward at the hips so your torso is parallel to the floor and your arms are perpendicular to your torso.
- Turn your shoulders 90 degrees to the left, so the fingers of your right hand point to (or actually touch) the floor and the fingers of your left hand point to the ceiling. Your arms should form a straight line.

- Keep your legs straight, and follow your top hand with your eyes.
- Turn back to the starting position, and then rotate your shoulders 90 degrees to the right.

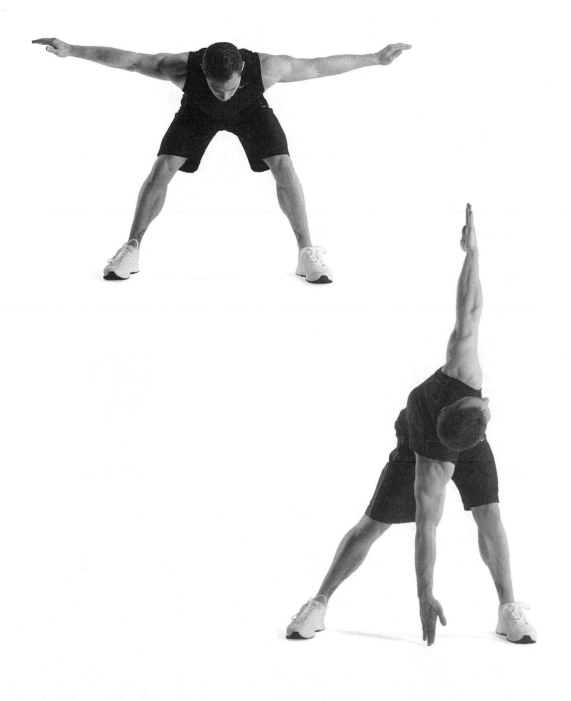

✳ Squat to Stand

- Stand with your hands at your sides and your feet shoulder-width apart.
- Bend at the hips, keeping your legs straight, and either grab, touch, or reach toward your toes, depending on your flexibility.
- Push your hips back, bend your knees, and grab your toes (if you haven't already) as you descend into a squat. Your arms remain straight and just inside your knees, and your feet absolutely must remain flat on the floor.
- Still holding your toes, pull your shoulders back and lift your head, as if you were in the bottom position of a barbell squat. Your feet are still flat on the floor.
- Raise your arms in a V shape toward the ceiling.
- Stand up. If you were at a wedding reception, you'd now be the Y in YMCA.
- Immediately bend at the hips and reach to your toes to start the next rep.

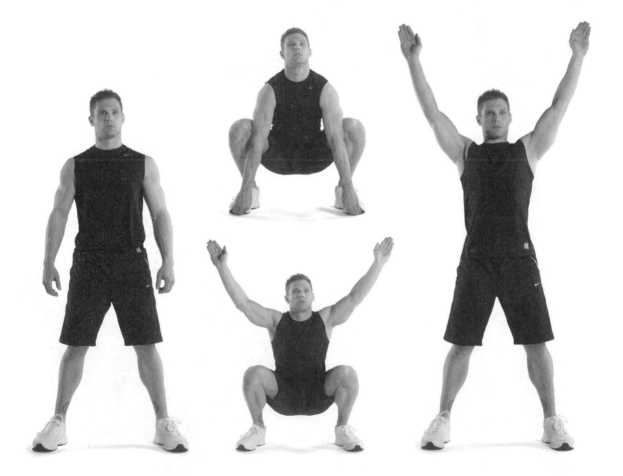

✳ Forward-Backward Jump

- Stand with your feet together, with your hips, knees, and ankles all bent slightly.
- Jump forward a couple inches with both feet, landing on your toes, and then immediately jump backward a couple inches.
- Continue until you finish 10 reps each direction, keeping your hips, knees, and ankles loose and "soft" to absorb impact. You shouldn't feel any jarring in your back or knees.

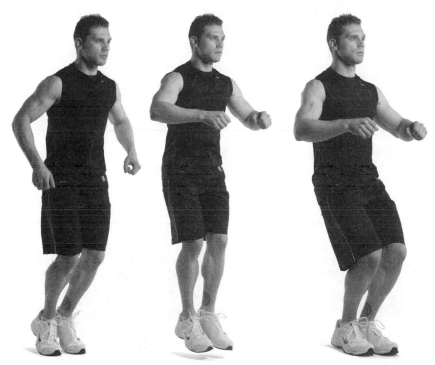

✳ Crossover Walking Toe Touch

- Stand with your feet hip-width apart.
- Take 3 steps forward—left, right, left—and after the third step, cross your right leg over your left, with both feet flat on the floor.
- Keeping both legs straight (or relatively straight), bend at the hips and reach down to or toward your toes.
- Feel the stretch in your hamstrings and calves, and straighten up.

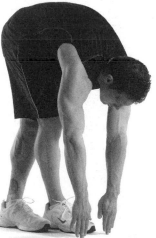

- Do three more steps—right, left, right—and after the third step, cross your left leg over your right, and repeat the reach and stretch.
- Continue for 10 to 20 yards.

✳ No-Space Option:

- Cross your right leg over your left, bend, and stretch.
- Come up, cross your left leg over your right, and repeat the stretch.
- Continue for 10 reps with each leg.

✳ Lateral Jump

- Stand with your feet together, with your hips, knees, and ankles all bent slightly.
- Jump a couple inches to your left with both feet, landing on your toes, and then immediately jump back to your right a couple inches.
- Do 10 reps each direction, keeping your hips, knees, and ankles "soft" to absorb impact.

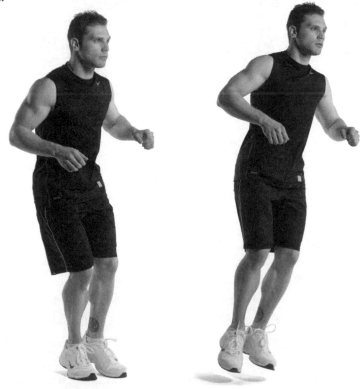

✳ Lateral Cross-Behind Lunge

- Stand with your feet shoulder-width apart and your hands in front of your chest or at your sides.
- Take a long step to your left, keeping your left toes pointed straight ahead, and drop into a side lunge, with your left knee bent 90 degrees, your right leg straight, and your torso upright.
- Rise out of the lunge, keeping your feet where they are, and then cross behind your left foot with your right.
- Step to your left and drop into another side lunge, rise, and cross behind again.
- Continue for 10 to 20 yards, then repeat to your right so you end up at your original spot.

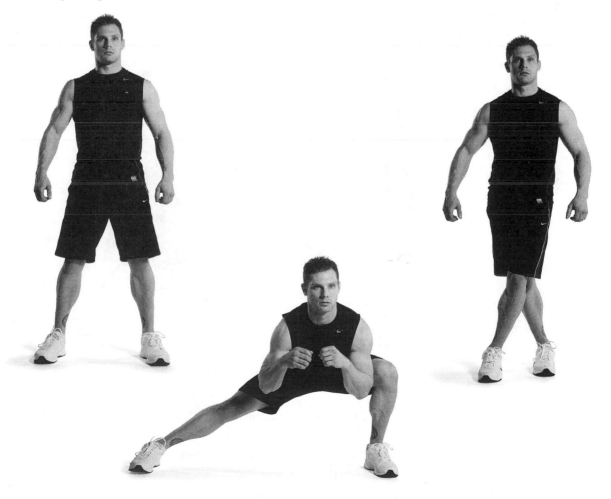

✳ No-space option:

- Do one lateral cross-behind lunge to your left, then do one back to your right.
- Alternate until you've done 10 side lunges in each direction.

✳ Seal Jack

- Stand with your feet together, arms straight out to your sides.
- Jump to spread your feet out wide as you bring your hands together in front of your chest. Keep your arms and legs straight.
- Jump back to the starting position.
- This is just like a jumping jack, only instead of bringing your hands together over your head, you do this in front of your torso. The modification helps warm up your chest and shoulder muscles before resistance exercises.

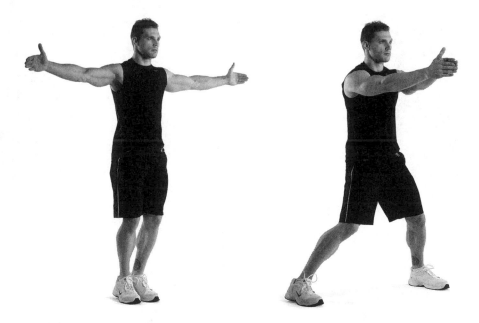

✳ Reverse Inchworm

- Stand with your back toward your destination, with your feet together and arms at your sides.
- Bend at the hips and reach toward the floor. Bend your knees as much as you must to put your palms on the floor.

- Take a long step back with each leg, putting you in the push-up position.
- Walk your toes backward until your hands are as far in front of your shoulders as you can manage without your lower back slipping out of the neutral position.
- Hold in that fully elongated position for a second, then walk your hands back to your feet until you can stand up.
- Rise to a full stand, then immediately bend at the hips to begin the next rep.

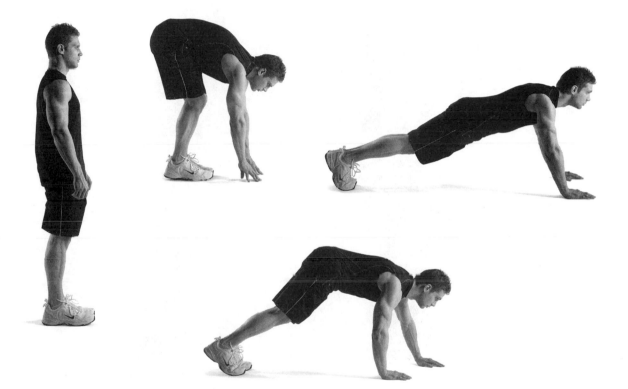

✳ **No-space option:**

- Alternate between forward and reverse inchworms: Start with the traditional inchworm exercise, in which you walk your hands forward to get into the fully extended position, then walk your toes forward to meet your hands. Do a reverse inchworm to get back to the starting position.
- Alternate until you've done 5 each way.

✳ Forward-Backward Hop

- This is the single-leg version of the forward-backward jump described earlier.
- Standing on your left foot, hop a few inches forward and a few inches back 10 times.
- Switch legs and repeat, hopping 10 times forward and back with your right foot.

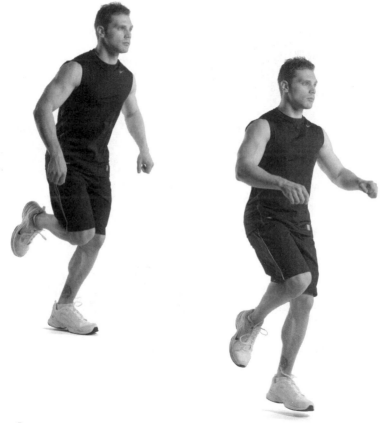

✳ Curtsy Lunge

- Stand with your feet shoulder-width apart and your hands together at your chest.
- Step behind and around your left leg with your right. Both sets of toes should point forward. Your feet probably will be 18 to 24 inches apart, with your right toes more or less on the same line as your left heel.
- Push your hips back and drop into a lunge, keeping your torso upright and shoulders square.
- Push down with your left heel to rise out of the lunge.

- Take a long step to the left with your left foot. Step behind again with your right foot, and drop into the next lunge.
- Do 5 curtsy lunges in this direction, then 5 lunges back to your starting spot, with your left leg reaching behind and around your right.

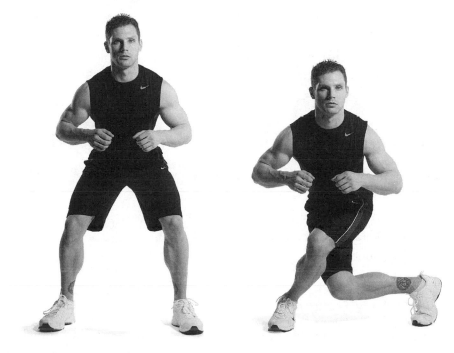

✳ No-space option:

- Alternate curtsy lunges to the left and right within the same space.

MOVEMENT SKILLS

The next three exercises are in a category called "movement skills." They're taken straight from athletic training, and are commonly used to warm up athletes in team and individual sports. You'll do each two times. You can do them consecutively, with a short rest in between, or in a circuit, in which you do each once and then repeat all three.

✳ Straight-Leg Skip

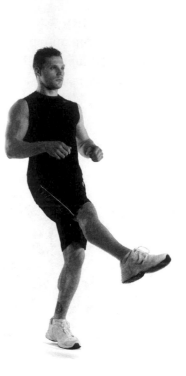

- Lean back slightly as you skip forward with your knees straight and your arms moving in rhythm with your legs.
- Go 10 to 20 yards, rest for a few seconds, and repeat.
- Another name for this might be the "drum-major skip." You want to catch a little air on each step.

✳ No-Space Option:

- Stand with your right hand resting on something sturdy for balance.
- Swing your left leg forward and back 10 times, keeping your knee straight but not locked.
- Repeat with your right leg.

✳ Social-Anxiety Option:

- Alwyn included the straight-leg skip because he wants you to do straight-leg skips. But we all realize that this is a very odd-looking thing to do outside the context of a team practice in which a bunch of people are doing the same exercise on instructions from a coach.
- So, if you have a space that allows you to go forward at least 10 yards, but just can't bring yourself to do straight-leg skips in the middle of a crowded health club, you can substitute walking high kicks. Kick your left foot up to touch your right hand, then your right foot up to meet your left hand.
- Go forward 10 to 20 yards, rest for a few seconds, and repeat.

✳ Side Shuffle with Arm Cross

- Get into a modified athletic position, with your feet wider than your shoulders, toes pointed forward, hips back, knees bent, torso leaning forward, arms out to your sides.

- Slide your right foot until it touches your left, simultaneously crossing your arms in front of your chest.
- Immediately step to the left with your left foot as you pull your arms back, then repeat the slide and arm cross.
- Go 10 to 20 yards to your left, rest for a few seconds, then shuffle back to your right.

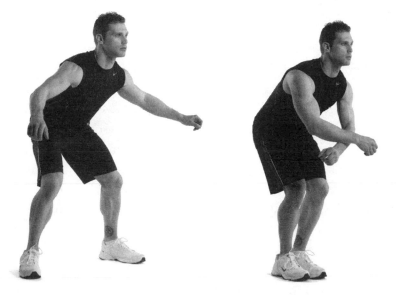

✳ Limited-Space and/or Social-Anxiety Option:

- Shuffle twice to your left, touching the floor just outside your left foot.
- Immediately change directions and shuffle to your right, touching the ground just beyond your right foot.
- Go 10 times each direction, then rest and repeat.
- This may look different from what others are doing, but nobody will look at you and wonder what you're up to. This lateral-movement pattern has applications in every sport that involves kicking, throwing, catching, or hitting a ball.

✳ Butt Kick

- Jog forward 10 to 20 yards, taking short steps and kicking yourself in the buttock with one heel on every step.

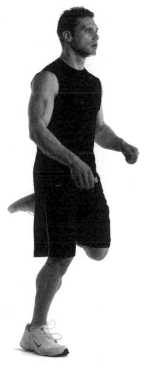

✳ Limited-Space and/or Social-Anxiety Option:

- Walk forward, pulling your heel to your butt with your same-side hand on each step.

ROLL YOUR OWN

Until I edited a book called *Core Performance*, by Mark Verstegen and Pete Williams, I'd never seen or even heard of foam-rolling exercises. They were among dozens of novel exercises included in *CP*, which I got a chance to try out in early 2003 on a visit to Athletes' Performance, Mark's facility in Tempe, Arizona. We broke out the rollers—6-inch-thick cylinders of unforgivingly dense foam—right after our strength workout. The experience was . . . unpleasant. I yelped in pain more than a few times.

I didn't realize that the discomfort was a sign that my lower-body muscles and connective tissues were much tighter than they should've been, setting me up for the injuries that came a few years later. My physical therapist included foam-rolling exercises in my rehab program. I'm convinced that those exercises, however uncomfortable they were at first, were just as important to my recovery as the dynamic warm-up and core training.

Technically, this type of training is called "myofascial self-release," and if you think of it in that context—breaking up the adhesions in your muscles and connective tissues that build up over time—it's a lot easier to convince yourself to take the plunge and include these exercises in your workouts.

I do them as part of my warm-up, but you don't have to. After your workout is fine. Or you can do them any other time of the day. You don't have to worry about preparing your body; just get down on the floor and roll.

There's no one routine that everyone has to follow, and no single technique. You can focus on your problem areas first, or start by loosening up surrounding tissues before you hit the tight spots. Use as much or as little pressure as you want. This is DIY training. It's a good idea to do some traditional stretches for your lower-body muscles after foam rolling, but it's not a requirement.

If your gym doesn't have foam rollers, or you work out at home, you can pick one up at a sporting-goods store, or order a three-foot-long roll from performbetter.com for $20 plus shipping. You can also do the exercises using a tennis ball for your calves and a basketball for bigger muscles like hamstrings and quadriceps.

✳ Back Roll

- Lie on the floor with the roll under the middle of your back.
- With your heels on the floor, pull and push your body over the roll, hitting your lower and middle back.
- You can also work your lower, middle, and upper back separately.

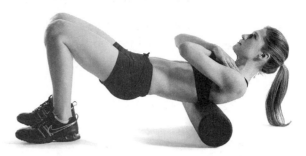

✳ Calf Roll

- Set the roll under one calf, and cross the ankle of your nonworking leg over that shin to increase the pressure.
- Lift your hips, supporting your weight on your hands, and pull and push your calf muscles over the roll from ankle to knee.
- Switch legs and repeat.

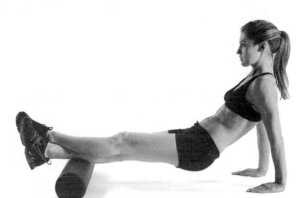

✳ Ham Roll

- Same technique as the calf roll, except now you roll from the bottom of your knee to the gluteal crease.
- Personally, I think it's kind of fun to propel myself back and forth over the roll when I work on my hamstrings. The power is coming from the muscles surrounding the shoulder joints, but the core muscles pitch in.

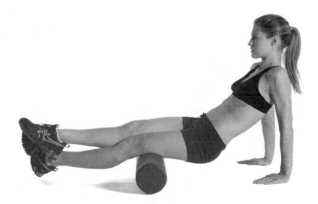

✳ Quad Roll

- This time you're facedown, with one or both of your front thighs on the roll and your weight on your forearms.
- Pull yourself over the roll, hitting everything from the top of your knee to your groin.

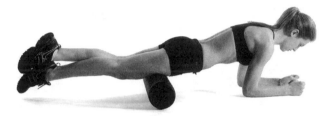

✳ IT-Band Roll

- Your iliotibial band is a sheath of connective tissue on the outside of your thigh. It starts at the top edge of your pelvis (the iliac crest), stretches over your abductor muscles, gets especially thick and tight alongside your thighbone, and ends just below your knee. The more you run, the tighter it'll get, since its job is to keep the bone inside the socket of your hip joint when all your weight is on one leg.
- Lie on your side, with the outside of your thigh on the roll and your weight on one hand.
- Pull and push yourself over the roll from your hip to the top of your knee.
- To take some pressure off, you can place the foot of your non-rolling leg on the floor.
- For most people foam rolling for the first time, this is an exercise that calls to mind the Spanish Inquisition. (For me it was the quad roll, probably from having done too many squats with too little soft-tissue work.) But the more it hurts, the more important it is to break up the adhesions making the area so tight and unyielding.

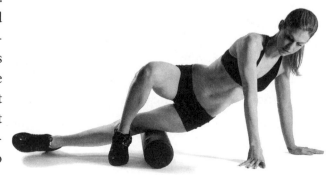

Strength: Phase One

10

Do EACH WORKOUT—A and B—at least six times, and as many as eight times. I don't think anybody who does this program will be familiar with all eight of the strength exercises, so the first week or two will be humbling for everyone; it's exactly what Alwyn had in mind. That said, if you're unfamiliar with *most* of the exercises, feel free to extend the program a little longer. It should take most readers four to eight weeks to complete Phase One.

Start each workout with the dynamic warm-up exercises shown in Chapter 9. (It's a good idea to finish the workout with the foam-rolling exercises shown at the end of Chapter 9, but it's not an official component of the program.) Train two to three times a week, with at least one full day off in between workout days.

Since there's no metabolic training at the end, these workouts should take about forty minutes to complete, once you're familiar with the exercises. You can add any type of non-strength-training exercise you want at the end, although it's not required.

WORKOUT A

Core: Stabilization

Exercise	Sets	Duration (seconds)	Rest (seconds)
1a: Plank	2	60–90	45–60
1b: Side plank	2 (each side)	30–45	45–60

For exercise descriptions, see Chapter 5.

Strength

Exercise	Sets	Reps	Rest (seconds)
1a: Split squat, front foot elevated	2–3	12 (each leg)	45–60
1b: Inverted row	2–3	12	45–60
2a: Romanian deadlift	2–3	12	45–60
2b: Push-up	2–3	12	45–60

WORKOUT B

Core: Stabilization

Exercise	Sets	Duration (seconds)	Rest (seconds)
1: Anti-rotation static hold	2	30 (each side)	45–60
2: Elevated plank	10	10	NA*
3: Elevated side plank	5	10 (each side)	NA*

*Relax for a second or two between sets, and a minute between exercises.

For exercise descriptions, see Chapter 5.

Strength

Exercise	Sets	Reps	Rest (seconds)
1a: Dumbbell single-leg Romanian deadlift	2–3	12 (each leg)	45–60
1b: Dumbbell alternating shoulder press*	2–3	12 (each arm)	45–60
2a: Overhead squat	2–3	12	45–60
2b: Cable kneeling pulldown	2–3	12	45–60

*Nonworking arm remains extended overhead.

STRENGTH EXERCISES

✳ Split Squat, Front Foot Elevated

GET READY

- You'll need a low step or box (I recommend no higher than 6 inches) and a pair of dumbbells (start light).
- Hold the dumbbells at arm's length at your sides.
- Start with your nondominant foot (your left if you're right-handed) on the box. Take a long step back with your other foot, as you would in a lunge.

MOVE

- Lower yourself until the thigh of your front leg is parallel to the floor.
- Push back up to the starting position.
- Do all your reps with your nondominant leg, then switch legs and repeat the set.

VARIATIONS

- It's much, much harder to do this with a barbell across the back of your shoulders.
- It might be a bit easier to do it while holding a weight plate across your chest with both hands.
- You can also hold a weight plate directly overhead. Whether this is easier or harder depends on how much weight you use on the dumbbell or barbell versions.

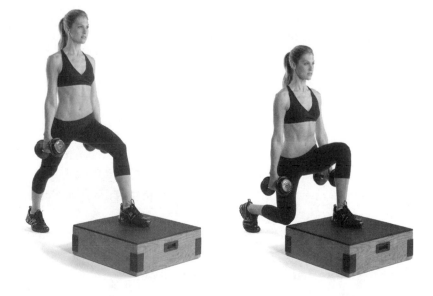

Obviously, holding a 45-pound plate overhead is easier than doing the exercise with two 45-pound dumbbells, or a 95-pound barbell.

CORE CHALLENGE

- This is considered a "posterior chain" exercise, meaning that your hamstrings and glutes function as the prime movers. But you should feel it in your entire lower body, including quadriceps, inner thighs, outer hips, and possibly even your calves. It really depends on how good your balance is; those with the worst balance will probably feel it most in muscles other than the prime movers.
- The stabilizer muscles in your core will fire to keep you upright. The barbell version will make those muscles work harder.

✳ Inverted Row

GET READY

- If you work out in a gym, it's easiest to do this with a Smith machine. Set the bar at a height that allows you to hang from it with your arms straight and your upper body off the floor. The higher you set the bar, the easier the exercise will be.
- If you work out at home, or in a gym that doesn't have a Smith machine, set a barbell on the supports of a squat rack, or anywhere else that's level, secure, and high enough off the floor to allow you to do the exercise.
- Grab the bar overhand, with your hands just beyond shoulder-width—whatever you'd use for a barbell bench press.
- Hang from the bar with straight arms and your heels on the floor. Your body should form a straight line from neck to ankles.

MOVE

- Pull your chest to the bar.
- Lower yourself to the starting position, and repeat.

VARIATIONS

- When you can't lower the bar any farther, you can make it harder by elevating your feet on a bench or Swiss ball.
- You can also raise one foot off the floor, which makes the core challenge much more intense.
- You'll sometimes see people do this with both feet flat on the floor and their knees bent. That makes it much easier, but also takes away much of the core challenge. It's better to go with a higher bar and straight legs.

CORE CHALLENGE

- New Rule #6 says that the lats are part of the core. Here's an exercise in which they work together. Rows work all the muscles in your upper and middle back as prime movers: lats, trapezius, rear shoulders. But when you do this with your body straight—no bend in your hips—your lats also work with your glutes as core stabilizers.

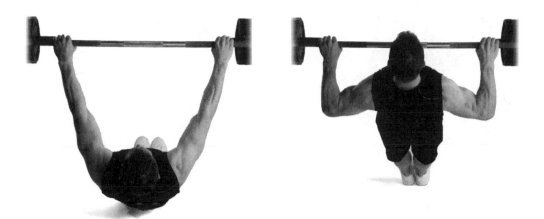

Alternative

✴ Suspended Row

- Attach a suspension trainer—TRX or equivalent—from a chin-up bar, and adjust the length to allow you to hang with straight arms with your heels on the floor and your body aligned from your ankles to your neck.
- Pull yourself up as far as you can while keeping your body straight.
- You can make the exercise harder by lowering the handles, or easier by raising them.
- You can use all the variations described above—feet elevated on a bench or Swiss ball, or with one foot lifted off the floor, bench, or ball.

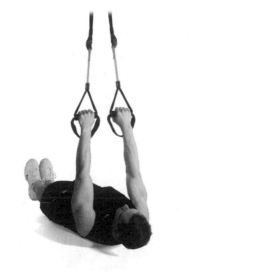
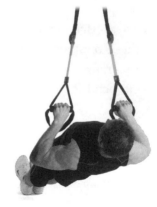

✳ Romanian Deadlift

GET READY

- Grab a barbell with an overhand, shoulder-width grip.
- Stand straight with your feet about hip-width apart and the barbell at arm's length against the front of your thighs.

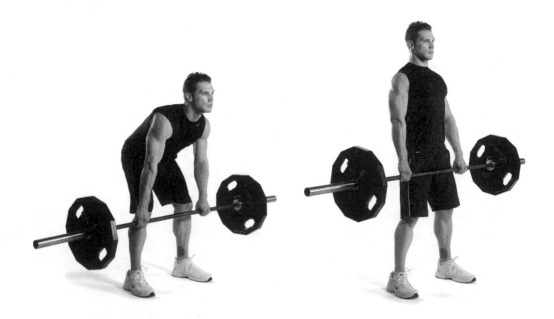

MOVE

- Push your hips back as you lower the bar until it's just below your knees. Your knees will bend a bit as your hips move back.
- Push your hips forward as you straighten your torso and pull the bar back to the starting position.

VARIATIONS

- You can also do this with dumbbells, although in this case it's really best to do it with a barbell unless one isn't available.

CORE CHALLENGE

- This is one of the best-known and most-used exercises for targeting the glutes and hamstrings, with the spinal erectors heavily involved to keep your lower back in the neutral position.

✴ Push-Up

GET READY

- Get down on the floor in the push-up position: arms straight down from your shoulders and perpendicular to the floor, weight resting on your hands and toes, your body in a straight line from neck to ankles.

MOVE

- Lower your chest to the floor.
- Push back up to the starting position.

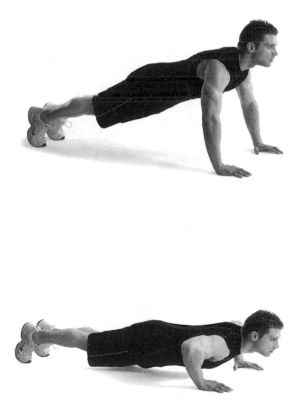

CORE CHALLENGE

- There's a reason why so many exercises in Chapters 5, 6, and 7 employ the push-up position. Simply holding that position activates all of your abdominal muscles. Lowering your chest to the floor and pushing back up again works your chest, front shoulders, and triceps, and increases the core challenge by virtue of the fact that your body is moving up and down.

Alternative #1

✳ Push-Up with Hands Elevated

- Traditionally, women who aren't yet strong enough to do regular push-ups are told to do the modified push-up, with knees on the floor. Alwyn won't let his female clients do this one because it drastically reduces the work for the core muscles. Instead, he likes the push-up with hands elevated. You still get the core challenge that comes with holding your body in the push-up position, but you can complete more reps with your upper body raised higher than your feet.

- Someone who's extremely deconditioned, or just coming back from a major illness or injury, could do this while standing and leaning forward to a wall.

- Others should choose an angle that allows them to do 12 reps on their first set and at least 10 on their second set. For women who're relatively new to lifting, you'll probably want to put your hands on a box that's about hip height (this would put your torso at a 45-degree angle to the floor, more or less), a box or bench that's about knee height (creating a 30-degree angle), or something in between.

- Your goal is to be able to do traditional push-ups; starting with this variation is fine, but you want to push yourself as aggressively as possible to increase upper-torso strength and lower the angle until you can do multiple sets of push-ups with your hands on the floor.

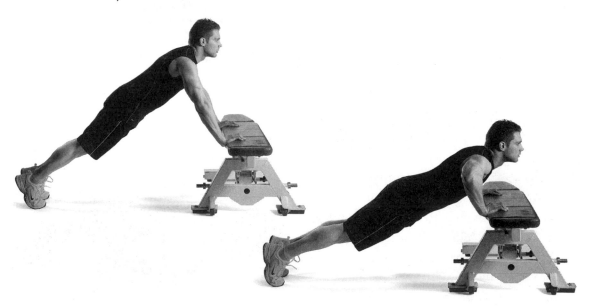

Alternative #2

✳ **Push-Up with Feet Elevated**

- This is the first variation for those looking to make the exercise more difficult, including most of the men doing Alwyn's workouts. If you can easily do three sets of 12 or more push-ups, make it harder by elevating your feet on a box or bench.
- Make this alternative harder by lifting one leg off the bench.

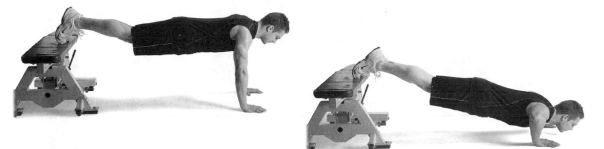

Alternative #3

✳ **Push-Up with Feet Elevated on Swiss Ball**

- Get into push-up position with your feet on a Swiss ball. Keep your body in a straight line from neck to ankles as you lower your chest to within a few inches of the floor, and then push back up again.
- It's a bit easier to do this with the tops of your feet and your shins on the ball, and a bit harder with your toes giving you the only points of contact with the ball.

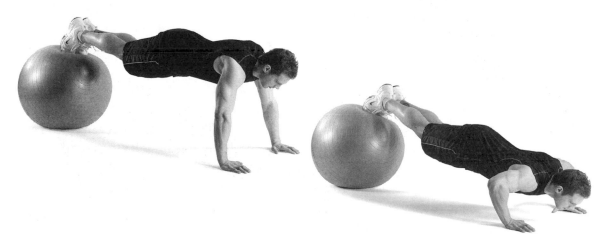

Alternative #4

✳ Push-Up with Feet Suspended

- Set up a TRX or equivalent so your feet are about 12 inches above the floor.
- Keep your body straight as you do push-ups with your feet in the suspension trainer.

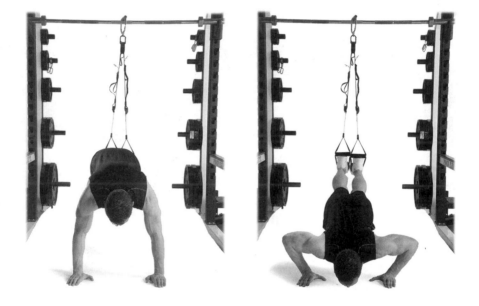

Alternative #5

✳ Push-Up with Hands on Bosu Ball

- Get a Bosu ball (it's the half-sphere on a solid plastic platform), and set it on the floor, ball-side down.
- Grab the outside edges of the platform, and get into push-up position.
- Lower your chest to the platform, then push back up to the starting position.
- You'll immediately feel a big difference from the other variations. Not only is it harder for your core muscles to keep you in alignment, it'll also be much more challenging for your chest and shoulder muscles. You're really doing stabilization training in two places: your core and your shoulders.
- The ultimate variation on a variation: try push-ups with your hands on a Bosu ball and your feet elevated on a bench.

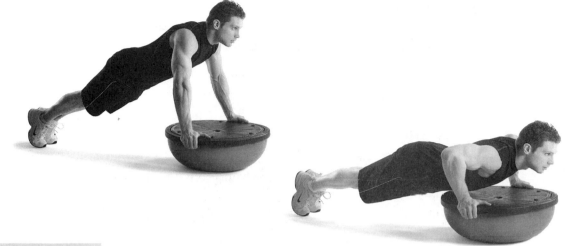

✳ Push-Up with Hands on Swiss Ball

- Get into push-up position with your hands on a Swiss ball. You'll have to play around with hand positions until you find the one that works best for you; it'll be a little different with bigger or smaller Swiss balls.
- Squeeze the ball with your hands as you lower your chest to the ball and then push back up again.
- This one is *really* hard to do. The stability challenge is so intense that you'll feel it immediately in your shoulders, triceps, chest, and abs.

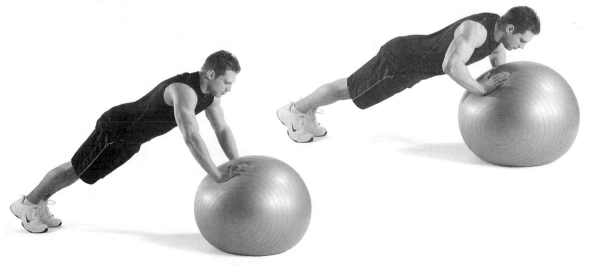

✳ Push-Up with Hands Suspended

- Although it took me a long time to get to it, this is the variation that Alwyn would like male readers to use, or to build up to.
- Set up a TRX or equivalent so your hands are about 12 to 24 inches above the floor. (Higher is easier, lower is harder.)
- Grab the handles and get into push-up position, with your arms straight and directly below your shoulders, and your body in a straight line from neck to ankles.

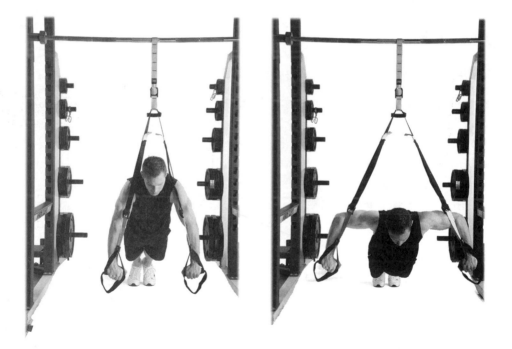

- Lower yourself until your chest is nearly at the level of your hands, then push back up to the starting position.
- In theory, you should be able to do this one with the exact same form you use for any other push-up variation. But in reality, your elbows probably will end up farther out from your torso than they are on non-suspended push-ups. That means a lot more work for your shoulders, and a much greater core challenge.

✳ T Push-Up

- Set up in push-up position.
- Lower yourself until your chest is close to the floor.
- As you push back up to the starting position, twist to your right, so your right arm ends up in the air straight over your left, and your body and arms form a T. Your weight will rest on your left hand and the outside edge of your left foot.
- Twist back and lower your right arm to the floor, then immediately begin the next push-up.
- At the top, twist to your left, so your left arm ends up in the air straight over your right. Twist back and immediately begin the next push-up.
- Each push-up, twisting to the left or the right, counts as one repetition. If you end one set on an odd number, start the next set with the side that did fewer reps.
- When you can do 12 reps in two consecutive sets, try it with one or two dumbbells the next time you do this workout. If you have hexagonal dumbbells, you can use two of them. Start with your hands on the dumbbells, and then do the exercise as described, alternating sides and lifting one of the dumbbells on each repetition.
- If you don't have hexagonal weights, you can use one round dumbbell. Start with one hand on the floor and the other on the dumbbell. Do a push-up, and as you come up, twist to the side with the weight, lifting it straight over-

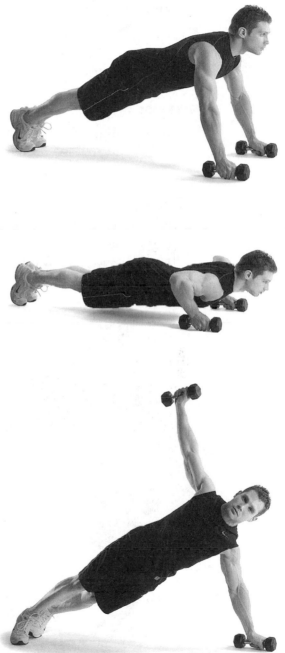

head. Do half your reps to that side (up to 6), then move the weight to the other hand and do the same number of reps, twisting to that side.

• The weighted versions of this exercise probably are the most difficult push-up variations you can do. The stronger you are, the heavier the weight you need to use to fatigue your muscles with 12 repetitions or less.

✳ Dumbbell Single-Leg Romanian Deadlift

GET READY

• Grab a dumbbell and hold it at arm's length in your right hand.
• Stand with your feet together.

MOVE

• Bend forward at the hips as you extend your right leg behind you, keeping your left leg straight or beat slightly at the knee. (Your left is the working leg in this part of the exercise.)
• Lower the weight toward the floor, with your right arm hanging straight down from your shoulder.

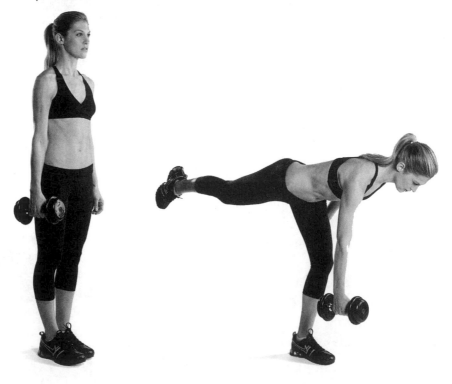

- Your body should be parallel to the floor, and form a straight line from your neck to your right ankle.
- Return to the starting position, and do all your reps (up to 12) standing on your left leg.
- Switch the weight to your left arm and repeat the set, extending your left leg behind you and standing on your right leg. (If you're left-handed, you probably want to start with the weight in your left hand, and work your right leg first.)

VARIATIONS

- You can also do this with two dumbbells, or even a barbell, but we don't recommend it. Using both arms at once creates more of a challenge for your upper-back muscles, and will induce a level of fatigue that makes it much harder to do the other strength exercises with full intensity and good form.

CORE CHALLENGE

- As with the Romanian deadlift described earlier, your glutes and hamstrings are the prime movers, with your spinal erectors working to keep your lower back in the neutral position. The balance component forces all the stabilizing muscles to make adjustments.

✳ Dumbbell Alternating Shoulder Press

GET READY

- Grab a pair of dumbbells and stand holding them at shoulder level, your palms turned toward each other.
- Raise the weight in your dominant arm straight up over your shoulder. You're going to hold it there as you do all your reps with your other arm.

MOVE

- Press the weight in your nondominant arm straight up over your shoulder.
- Lower it and repeat until you've done all your reps (up to 12).
- On the final rep, keep that arm straight, and lower the weight in your dominant arm.
- Do all your reps with your dominant arm while holding the weight in your nondominant arm straight up over your shoulder.

DON'T

- Lean backward toward the end of the set, as your trunk muscles fatigue. If you can't hold your posture and stay upright, end the set.

CORE CHALLENGE

- As I noted, the main challenge for your core is staying upright when your body wants to lean back.
- Honestly, though, that's a minor concern. The main benefit of this exercise comes from the astounding challenge to your shoulder stabilizers—the trapezius and all the other muscles that hold together the sometimes-fragile complex of bones that make up your shoulder girdle. The deltoids, the most visible shoulder muscles, will get an incredible workout, along with your triceps.

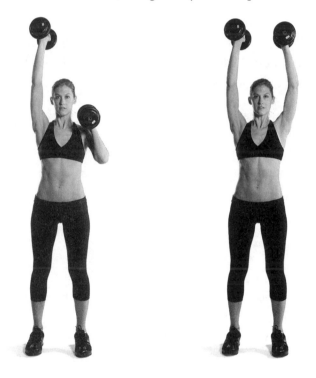

✴ Overhead Squat

GET READY

- You'll need something solid and straight to hold with both arms overhead. Most readers, male and female, won't be able to start with the 45-pound Olympic barbell, even without any weight plates added to it. Most women will want to start with a broomstick or plastic dowel rod, while men might start with a 10-pound standard barbell. (It's the one that uses plates with a one-inch hole in the middle, as opposed to the two-inch hole on Olympic plates.)

- If you have experience doing overhead squats, or training in the snatch, one of the two exercises contested in Olympic weight lifting, ignore the previous instructions, and use as much weight as you can handle.
- Stand with your feet shoulder-width apart, toes pointed straight ahead or angled out slightly.
- Grab the bar overhand with your hands about double shoulder width. Hold it over the back of your shoulders with your arms straight.

MOVE

- Push your hips back as you descend into a squat.
- Go as low as you can while keeping your arms straight and the bar over the back of your shoulders.
- Rise back to the starting position and repeat.

DON'T

- Allow your lower back to go into an excessive arch.
- Allow the bar to come forward, over your head. Your arms need to be perpendicular to the floor throughout the exercise.

CORE CHALLENGE

- This exercise is almost nothing but core challenge. The load isn't heavy, compared to what you could lift on a conventional squat. What's extremely hard is holding it overhead as you squat down and then stand up.

✳ Cable Kneeling Pulldown

GET READY

- Attach a long bar to the lat-pulldown station.
- Grab the bar with an overhand grip that's about one and a half times shoulder width.
- Rather than sit on the padded seat, kneel behind it. Get as close as you can without touching the seat with your abdomen or pelvis.

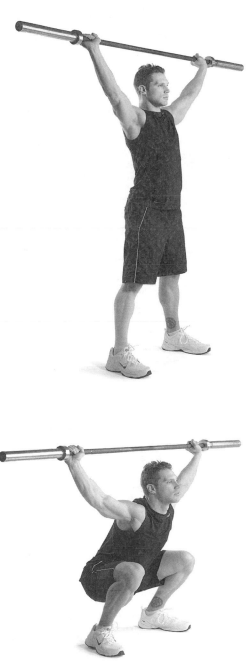

- Straighten your torso, square your shoulders, and hold the bar with your arms straight and angled slightly in front of your torso.

MOVE

- Pull the bar to your upper chest, pushing your chest out to meet it.
- Squeeze your shoulder blades together in back, and return the bar to the starting position.

DON'T

- Pull the bar down along the front of your torso. Pull it *to your chest*. I see women do this quite a bit, internally rotating their upper arms at the shoulder joints to pull it lower. If you can pull it lower than your chest, it's a sure sign that you're using too little weight, in addition to the problems with your technique.
- Pull the bar halfway down, or do half-reps by starting with your arms bent. I see men do this; often, it's the biggest, strongest guys. If you can't pull the bar to your chest, you're using too much weight to get all the benefits of the exercise. Don't worry if you pull the bar to your chest on 10 reps but only get halfway on the 11th. You did every complete repetition possible—a damned good set. End the set there. If you don't get at least 10 or 11 full-range-of-motion reps on your first set, it's a sign that you were too aggressive and need to use less weight. If you get

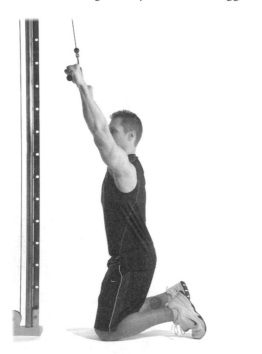
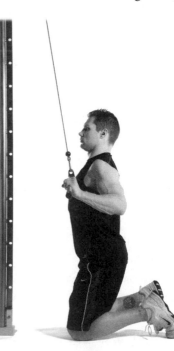

12 easily on that first set, and feel you could've gotten 3 or 4 more, use more weight on the next set. Whatever weight you choose, you want to make sure you get most of the reps with perfect form.

CORE CHALLENGE

- This is another exercise that uses the lats as prime movers while simultaneously using the lats and glutes for core stability. When you sit to do pulldowns, your glutes are in a stretched position, preventing them from working with your lats to support your lumbar spine. Granted, your lower back isn't in danger in that position, but that's not the point. You want to train those muscles to support your back when there's little chance of injury, so they help you out when there is a risk.

11

Strength: Phase Two

IN THIS PHASE you're going to use heavier weights for fewer reps and more sets. You won't have to work as hard on balance as you did in Phase One, allowing you to be more aggressive with your weight selection. (You also have the option of adding a basic, heavy lift to each workout, which I'll explain at the end of the chapter.)

Start each workout with the mobility exercises in Chapter 9. You'll finish each workout with 10 to 20 minutes of metabolic training, shown in this chapter.

As with Phase One, you'll do workouts A and B six to eight times each. It should take you four to eight weeks to finish Phase Two.

WORKOUT A

Core: Dynamic Stabilization			
Exercise	Sets	Reps	Rest (seconds)
1: Valslide push-away	1	10–12	60–90
2: Swiss-ball mountain climber	1	10–12 (each leg)*	60–90
3: Cable half-kneeling chop	1	10–12 (each side)†	60–90

*Do slow reps at first, then progress by speeding up movement.
†Do slow reps, and progress by adding weight.
 For exercise descriptions, see Chapter 6.

Strength			
Exercise	Sets	Reps	Rest (seconds)
1a: Dumbbell split squat	3–4	8 (each leg)	60–90
1b: Dumbbell two-point row	3–4	8 (each arm)	60–90
2a: Wide-grip deadlift with feet on weight plate	3–4	8	60–90
2b: Dumbbell alternating chest press on partial bench	3–4	8 (each arm)	60–90

Metabolic

For 10 minutes, do 6 to 10 burpees per minute. You should spend 20 to 30 seconds doing the burpees, and then rest until it's time to start the next set. Your work-to-rest ratio, thus, should be between 1-to-1 and 1-to-2. Add one set (one minute, 6 to 10 burpees) each week. Sometimes you'll do Workout A twice a week, and sometimes you'll only do it once. Add just one set per week to your metabolic training no matter how many times you do the workout in any given week.

WORKOUT B

Core: Dynamic Stabilization			
Exercise	Sets	Reps	Rest (seconds)
1: Front plank and pulldown	1	10–12 (each arm)	60–90
2: Side plank and row	1	10–12 (each arm)	60–90
3: Swiss-ball jackknife	1	10–12	60–90
4: Cable kneeling cross-body lift	1	10–12 (each side)	60–90
For exercise descriptions, see Chapter 6.			

Strength			
Exercise	Sets	Reps	Rest (seconds)
1a: Dumbbell step-up	3–4	8 (each leg)	60–90
1b: Dumbbell one-arm push press	3–4	8 (each arm)	60–90
2a: Dumbbell offloaded front squat	2*	8	60–90
2b: Mixed-grip chin-up	2†	8	60–90
*Switch sides with the weights for the second set.			
†Reverse your grip for the second set.			

Metabolic

For 10 minutes, do 10 to 12 kettlebell or dumbbell swings per minute. You should spend 20 to 30 seconds doing the swings, and then rest until it's time to start the next set. Your work-to-rest ratio, thus, should be between 1-to-1 and 1-to-2. Add one set (one minute, 10 to 12 swings) each week. Sometimes you'll do Workout B twice a week, and sometimes you'll only do it once. Add just one set per week to your metabolic training no matter how many times you do the workout in any given week.

STRENGTH EXERCISES

✳ Dumbbell Split Squat

GET READY

- Grab a pair of relatively heavy dumbbells, and hold them at arm's length at your sides.

- Stand with your feet hip-width apart, and then take a long step back with your dominant leg, so your nondominant leg is in front.

MOVE
- Lower your body until the top of your front thigh is parallel to the floor and your rear knee nearly touches the floor.
- Push back to the starting position.
- Do all your reps (up to 8), then switch legs and repeat the set.

CORE CHALLENGE
- You're working all your lower-body muscles, while your core muscles fire to keep your torso upright.

VARIATION
- You can also do this with one dumbbell instead of two. Hold the dumbbell with the hand opposite the front leg. So if your left leg is in front, hold the weight with your right hand.

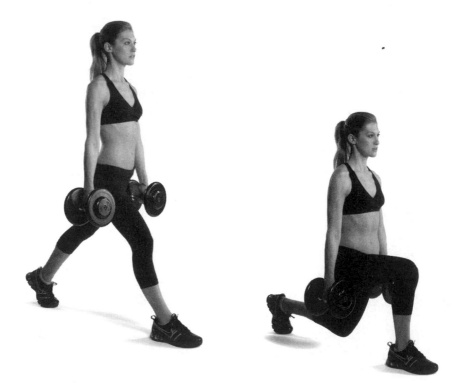

✴ Dumbbell Two-Point Row

GET READY

- Grab a dumbbell and hold it in your nondominant hand.
- Stand with your feet shoulder-width apart, knees bent slightly.
- Push your hips back as you bend your torso forward.
- Hold the weight straight down from your shoulder with an overhand grip (palm facing back).

MOVE

- Pull the weight straight up to the side of your abdomen.
- Finish all the reps (up to 8), then repeat the set with the other arm.

CORE CHALLENGE

- With your torso bent forward from the hips, your spinal stabilizers have to work hard to keep your lower back in the neutral position. Using one arm at a time increases this challenge.

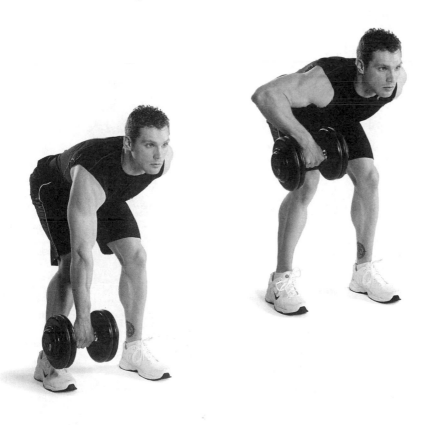

✳ Wide-Grip Deadlift with Feet on Weight Plate

GET READY

- Load a barbell and set it on the floor in front of a 45-pound weight plate, which is placed on the floor with the lettered side down.
- Stand on the plate with your feet shoulder-width apart and toes pointed forward.
- Squat and grab the bar overhand with a double-shoulder-width grip. Roll the bar to your toes.
- Tighten up your body and your grip. You want your hips back, knees bent, chest over your thighs, arms straight, shoulders square, eyes forward.

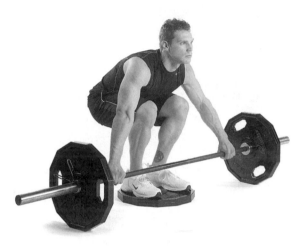

MOVE

- Stand and pull the bar straight up your shins.
- Once the bar is past your knees, push your hips forward and pull your shoulder blades together in back to complete the lift.
- Lower it the floor and repeat.

CORE CHALLENGE

- This is one of Alwyn's favorite and most effective exercises for training thighs, hips, and shoulders, with a tremendous challenge to the muscles supporting your upper back and to those stabilizing your lumbar spine. By standing on a weight

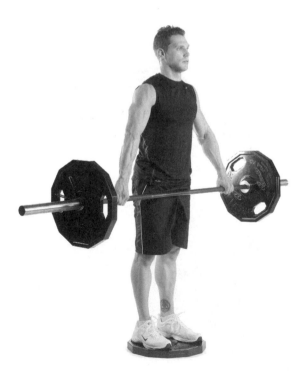

plate, you're adding an extra inch to the range of motion, creating more work for your hamstrings and glutes (and a bit more for your quads than you'd ordinarily get on a deadlift). And by using a wide grip you're increasing the challenge to your trapezius and the other muscles surrounding your shoulder blades.

✳ Dumbbell Alternating Chest Press on Partial Bench

GET READY

- You'll need a pair of moderately heavy dumbbells and a bench.
- Lay your head and shoulders at one end of a flat bench, with your torso and legs extending from it. Everything from your middle back to your feet is unsupported.
- Set your feet flat on the floor, shoulder-width apart.
- Tighten up your body so it forms a straight line from your knees through your neck.
- Hold the weights at the sides of your chest; the outside edges of the dumbbells should be a couple inches beyond your pectoral muscles (obviously, a lot depends on the size of the weights), and just below your shoulders.

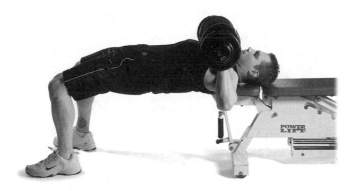

MOVE

- Press the weight with your nondominant arm until your arm is straight, lower it, and then press the other. That's one repetition. Alternate until you do all the reps (up to 8) with each arm.

CORE CHALLENGE

- Your chest, front shoulders, and triceps are the prime movers. But with your body hanging off in space and only your shoulders supported on the bench, you're activating all the muscles in your hips and torso that work to stabilize your spine.

VARIATION

- If you want an even more intense core challenge, try using one dumbbell at a time. Start with your nondominant arm, with your dominant hand resting on your abdomen. Do all your reps, then switch arms and repeat. You can feel your abdominal muscles working hard on both sides of your torso.

✳ Dumbbell Step-Up

GET READY

- Grab a pair of dumbbells and stand in front of a step or bench. A higher step is harder and calls for more modest weights, while a lower step allows you to go heavier through a shorter range of motion.
- Place the foot of your nondominant leg flat on the step.

MOVE

- Push down through the heel of the foot on the step and lift yourself so your trailing leg is even with your working leg.
- Brush the step with your nonworking foot—don't put any weight on it while it's on the step—and then lower that foot to the starting position.
- Do all your reps (up to 8) with your nondominant leg, then switch legs and repeat the set.

DON'T

- Push off the floor with your trailing foot. You want all the force generated by the leg that's on the step. The more fatigued you are, the harder it is to resist the temptation to give yourself a boost with your back leg.

CORE CHALLENGE

- Your prime movers are the hamstrings and glutes of your working leg, with contributions from your calves and quadriceps. One reason I've always liked this exercise is that you can feel other muscles coming into play as the supporting muscles in your calves, thighs, and hips start to fatigue. Of course, your core muscles work to keep you upright, and that challenge also changes as muscles get tired and you have to work harder to keep your balance.

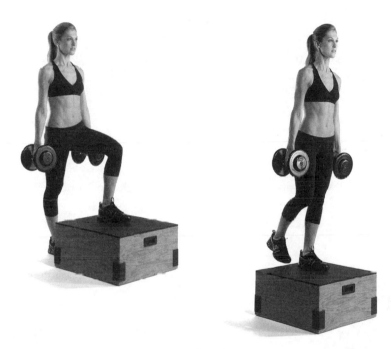

VARIATIONS

- There are lots of different ways to do step-ups to increase the core challenge—holding a barbell across the back of your shoulders makes the exercise much harder, and you can change things up by holding weights overhead. Those are terrific exercises, but if you do them with the first exercise, you'll create too much fatigue in muscles that you'll need later in the workout. If you want to progress beyond the plain-vanilla dumbbell version shown here, you can try step-ups with one weight instead of two. Hold the dumbbell in your right hand if you're stepping up with your left leg, and vice versa.

✳ Dumbbell One-Arm Push Press

GET READY

- Grab a moderately heavy dumbbell with your nondominant hand and stand holding it alongside your shoulder with your feet shoulder-width apart.

MOVE

- Bend at the knees and hips, as if you were about to jump.
- As you snap your hips forward and straighten your knees, use that momentum to push the weight straight up from your shoulder.
- Lower the weight to your shoulder, and immediately dip again and repeat.
- Finish all your reps (up to 8) with your nondominant arm, then switch and repeat the set.

DON'T

- Be timid. As soon as you feel comfortable with the exercise, push yourself aggressively to use heavier weights. Power exercises like this one are a lot of fun to do, especially if you've done most of your lifting with moderate weights and slow,

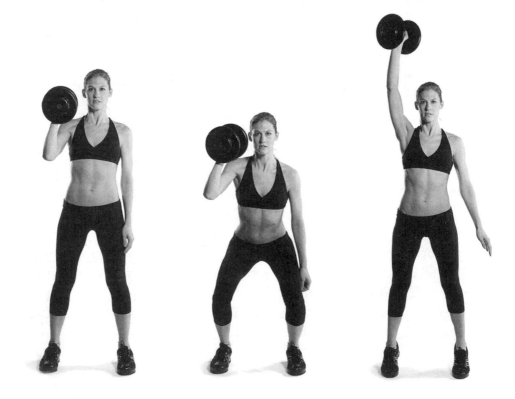

careful execution. You can really move fast and explosively with the push press, and use more weight than you've ever pressed overhead before.

CORE CHALLENGE

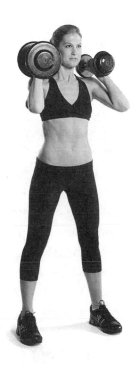

- Most people would look at this as a shoulder exercise with a "cheat" move: momentum generated by the lower body. But really it's a lower-body exercise with some shoulder and triceps action at the end. The power for the move comes from the extensor chain— glutes and hamstrings—with your core muscles acting as the conduit. That is, they help you transfer the power from those muscles to your shoulder and arm. Your hips also have a secondary role: Not only are they creating movement on the way up, they're absorbing impact as you come back down, in concert with your knees and ankles. If you were actually jumping with a weight in your hand, those muscles would have to soften the landing; without them bending as you land, your spine would have to take the brunt of the impact.

✴ Dumbbell Offloaded Front Squat

GET READY

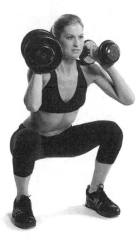

- Grab a pair of dumbbells of unequal weight. One should be about 10 pounds heavier than the other.
- Stand with your feet shoulder-width apart and toes pointed straight ahead or angled out slightly.
- Lift the weights to your shoulders with your palms facing each other and your elbows out in front of you.
- The edges of the dumbbells should rest on your shoulders.

MOVE

- Push your hips back as you lower yourself into a squat.
- Descend until the tops of your thighs are parallel to the floor, keeping your torso upright.
- Push back up to the starting position, then repeat until you complete all your reps (up to 8).
- For your second set, switch the weights, so the heavier one is on the opposite side.

CORE CHALLENGE

- Front squats work all your lower-body muscles, and your core has to work especially hard to keep your torso upright. Any forward lean will dislodge the weights from their perch on your shoulders, effectively ending your set. Combine that with unbalanced weights, and you have a full-spectrum core challenge: The spinal stabilizers work to keep your back in the neutral position; abdominal muscles squeeze your internal organs to create stabilizing pressure from the front; and the obliques and quadratus lumborum, the muscles controlling side-to-side movement, have to deal with the unequal distribution of the load.

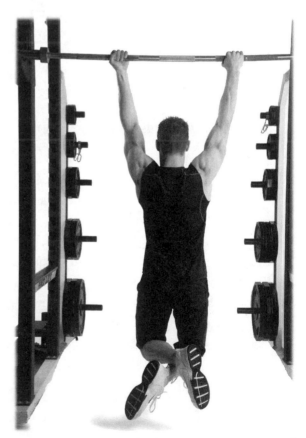

✳ Mixed-Grip Chin-Up

GET READY

- If you've done deadlifts with near-max weights, you've probably used the mixed grip: one hand under the bar, one hand over. It allows you to lift far more weight than you could with an overhand grip on both sides of the bar. This is the same idea: Instead of an overhand or underhand grip, grab the chin-up bar with a mixed grip, your hands just beyond shoulder-width apart.

- Hang from the bar with your arms straight.
- Bend your knees and cross your ankles in back. Your body should form a straight line from your wrists to your knees.

MOVE

- Pull your body up as high as you can, with your chin a couple inches over the bar.
- Lower yourself to the starting position, and finish all your reps (up to 8).
- For your next set, reverse the grip—whichever hand was over the bar goes under, and vice versa.

CORE CHALLENGE

- This is yet another exercise in which your lats act as prime movers while also working with your glutes to provide spinal stability. This time there's the additional challenge of the mixed grip. Your body will tend to rotate a bit toward the side with the underhand grip, and all your torso muscles will have to work to prevent that rotation.

ALTERNATIVE #1: Band-assisted mixed-grip chin-up

- If you can't do chin-ups, Alwyn recommends using an elastic band to help you move your body weight, as shown on page 161, lower left. Secure the band around the middle of the bar, and then put your knees through the loop at the bottom. The thicker the band, the more help you'll get, and the more reps you'll be able to do.

ALTERNATIVE #2: Kneeling mixed-grip lat pulldown

- This is a decidedly inferior option, since there won't be as much of an anti-rotation challenge when you're pulling a bar to your chest as opposed to pulling your chest up to a bar. But it's better than not doing the exercise at all. Set up as you would for the kneeling lat pulldown described in the previous chapter, only with a mixed grip. Use a challenging weight, and start each rep with an explosive pull, as you would if you were doing a chin-up.

METABOLIC EXERCISES

✳ Burpee

GET READY

- Stand on a carpeted or impact-absorbing wooden floor with your feet hip-width apart.
- Make sure you're facing a clock or holding or wearing a watch that tracks time to the second.
- When the second hand hits 12, start the exercise.

MOVE

- Squat down and put your hands on the floor outside your feet.
- Thrust your legs backward so you're in the push-up position.
- Pull your legs back in.
- Jump, thrusting your arms overhead and coming all the way up off the floor.
- As you land, immediately squat down for the next rep.
- Do 6 to 10 reps, then rest until the second hand hits 12 again.
- Do 6 to 10 reps every minute for 10 minutes the first week. Add one set—1 minute, 6 to 10 reps—every week until you finish the program.
- The goal is to achieve a 1-to-1 or 1-to-2 work-to-rest ratio—20 to 30 seconds of work and 30 to 40 seconds of rest before you begin the next set.

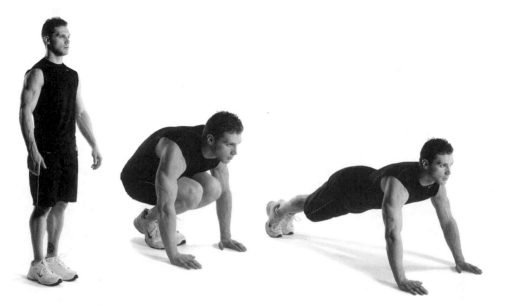

CORE CHALLENGE

- This exercise is a combination of two separate movements: squat thrust and vertical jump. (You can also do it with a push-up, but we don't recommend it here.) Both those exercises require core stability, but the real challenge is keeping your back in the neutral position as you deal with increasing fatigue.

✳ Dumbbell or Kettlebell Swing

GET READY

- Grab a kettlebell or dumbbell and hold it with both hands in front of your torso, with your arms straight.
- Set your feet wider than shoulder width, your toes pointed straight ahead or angled out slightly.
- As with the burpees, you need to be able to see a clock with a second hand. When it hits 12, start the set.

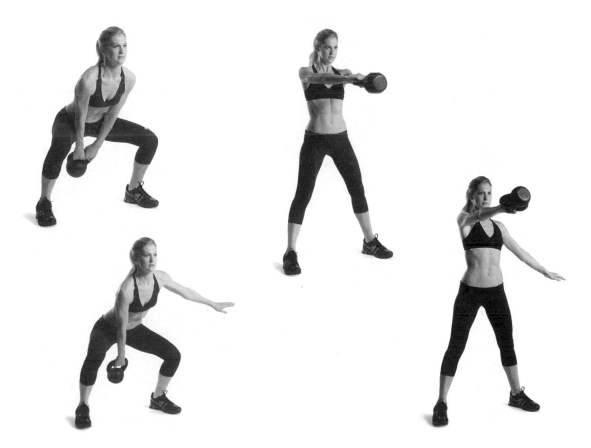

MOVE

- Push your hips back as you squat down, reaching as far back between your legs as you can.
- Snap your hips forward as you straighten your knees. Let the momentum of the hip thrust send the weight swinging upward to about chest height.
- As soon as the weight reaches the top of its trajectory, push your hips back again and let the weight swing back between your legs.
- Do 10 to 12 swings, and rest until the second hand hits 12 again.
- Do 10 to 12 reps every minute for 10 minutes the first week. Add one set— 1 minute, 10 to 12 reps—every week until you finish the program.

DON'T

- Pull the weight with your shoulder muscles. It's not a "shoulder" exercise like the front raise. You want all the power to come from your glutes and hamstrings.

CORE CHALLENGE

- Since your hip-straightening muscles are doing all the lifting, that means your spinal stabilizers are challenged on every rep to keep your back in the neutral position despite rapidly increasing fatigue.

VARIATION

- It's more fun to do this with one arm at a time. Alternate arms on each set.
- If you're using a kettlebell, you can switch hands on each rep, which certainly keeps you focused, if nothing else. You need to let go of the handle at the top of the trajectory, and grab it with your other hand. Alternate like this for 10 reps.
- If you're using a dumbbell, you can try the same thing, but I admit I've never tried it, and don't plan to. However, I have done a version of this exercise in which I let go of the weight halfway up, and then caught it with the same arm at the top of the trajectory. I don't recommend it, especially if you work out in a commercial gym, but I'd be lying if I said it wasn't fun to do.

EXTRA STRENGTH

Of the three phases, Phase Two is the most focused on strength and hypertrophy. The exercises are simpler than the ones in Phase One. They require less balance and coordination, allowing you to work with relatively heavy weights for as many as 4 sets of 8 repetitions.

But what do you do if you want to work with weights that aren't just *relatively* heavy? That's where Extra Strength comes in: If you're an intermediate to advanced lifter, you can add one heavy lift to the start of your strength training in each workout in Phase Two.

Here's how it works:

Right after your core training, you'll do one of these four exercises: front squat, deadlift, chin-up, shoulder press. Then you'll do the four exercises in the regular Phase Two workout. You want to do each of the Extra Strength exercises four times (I'll explain why in a moment), which means you'll do 16 total workouts. If you train three times a week, on a Monday-Wednesday-Friday schedule, a 16-workout program will look like this:

	Monday	Wednesday	Friday
Week 1	Workout A + front squat	Workout B + shoulder press	Workout A + chin-up
Week 2	Workout B + deadlift	Workout A + front squat	Workout B + shoulder press
Week 3	Workout A + chin-up	Workout B + deadlift	Workout A + front squat
Week 4	Workout B + shoulder press	Workout A + chin-up	Workout B + deadlift
Week 5	Workout A + front squat	Workout B + shoulder press	Workout A + chin-up
Week 6	Workout B + deadlift		

You'll use different reps each time you do each exercise. To keep this straight, we'll add a new term: *rotation*. One rotation is four workouts—two each of Workout A and Workout B—during which you do each Extra Strength exercise once.

The following chart shows the sets and reps you'll use on each rotation.

	Sets	Reps
Rotation 1	4	8,6,4,8
Rotation 2	4	7,5,3,7
Rotation 3	4	6,4,2,6
Rotation 4	4	5,3,1,5

The object is to use a heavier weight for each of the first three sets, then do a final set with a lighter weight. Let's say you're doing deadlifts. After a warm-up, you might use these weights:

Set	Reps	Weight (pounds)
1	8	185
2	6	205
3	4	225
4	8	205

As you can see, you use the same weight on the fourth set that you used on the second, but you do more reps—8 instead of 6. That means you leave a little in the tank on the first three sets and go all-out on that fourth set. It should feel a little lighter on the fourth set than it did on the second, since you used a heavier weight in between on the third set.

You increase the weights, and lower the reps, with each rotation. By the time you get to the fourth rotation, you should be working with much heavier weights than you were able to use before you started the Extra Strength program.

But here's the first complication: After you finish your Extra Strength exercise, you still have to do four more exercises to complete the workout. Those include variations of the Extra Strength exercises.

Let's use deadlifts as an example. You do a wide-grip deadlift standing on a weight plate in Workout A, and you do Workout A eight times in a 16-workout program. But you also do conventional deadlifts four times as part of Extra Strength. That means you'll do deadlifts a total of 12 times in 16 workouts. In Week 3, you'll do deadlifts in three consecutive training sessions. (If you follow the schedule I showed earlier, you'll never do both types of deadlift in the same workout.)

That's a lot of deadlifts. You may need to be cautious in Workout A, either by using somewhat lighter weights, or by doing three sets of deadlifts instead of four.

There's much less potential for overdoing it with the other exercises. You'll only do two sets of mixed-grip chin-ups and offloaded front squats in Workout B, which shouldn't conflict with your Extra Strength chin-ups and front squats (which you'll do on different days if you follow the schedule). If anything, the exercises probably will complement each other, with each increasing the training effect you get from the other without compromising recovery.

That brings me to the second complication: time. You need to do a specific warm-up for each Extra Strength exercise (I recommend at least two warm-up sets with lighter weights), and you need to rest longer in between sets—probably two to three minutes. Your workouts will go well past an hour if you do the entire program—10 minutes of dynamic mobility, 10 minutes of core training, 10 to 15 minutes of Extra Strength, 20 minutes of resistance training, and 10 to 20 minutes of metabolic work.

Something has to go, right? In this case, it's the metabolic training, and now we get into the issue of setting priorities. If you're already somewhat lean and most interested in adding strength and size, it's an easy call; you won't miss the metabolic work. But if you're a fairly advanced lifter who also has fat to lose, it's a tougher decision.

Let's start with a definition: If you've been lifting consistently for at least three to five years, you've experienced significant gains in strength and muscle size, and you're familiar with all four exercises in Extra Strength, you're an intermediate to advanced lifter. If you've never done deadlifts or front squats with heavy weights and low reps, this definition doesn't apply to you. No matter how much time you've spent in the gym, at best you're an intermediate. More likely, you're still a beginner, in terms of your training knowledge, strength, and skill.

An advanced lifter needs to use heavy weights at least some of the time to maintain strength, even if the goal is fat loss. So even without the metabolic work in Phase Two, you're still getting about an hour of serious training three times a week, which should improve your body composition.

But to make it come off faster, you can take the metabolic work from Phase Two and use it in Phase One. Then do Phase Two with Extra Strength but without the metabolic training. And finish with Phase Three exactly as written. Everyone will lose fat on that one.

EXTRA STRENGTH EXERCISES

✳ Front Squat

GET READY

- Set up a barbell in the squat rack at about shoulder height.
- Grab it with an overhand, shoulder-width grip, and rotate your arms upward until your upper arms are nearly parallel to the floor.
- Balance the bar on your front shoulders as you lift it off the supports. The bar will roll from your palms to your fingers as you balance it on your shoulders. As long as you keep your arms up and your torso upright, it'll stay in this spot.
- Step back from the rack and set your feet shoulder-width apart, with your toes pointed straight ahead or angled out slightly.

MOVE

- Push your hips back and lower your body until the tops of your thighs are parallel to the floor, or lower.
- Rise back to the starting position.

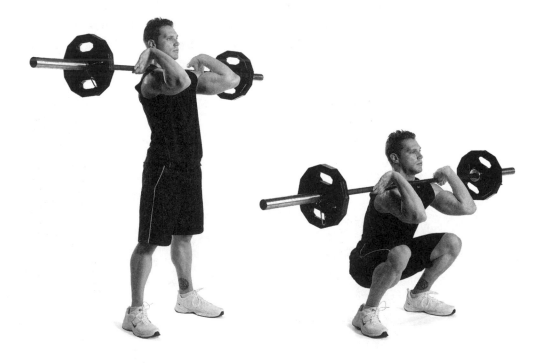

✴ Shoulder Press

GET READY

- Set up a barbell in the squat rack at about shoulder height.
- Grab the bar overhand with your hands wider than your shoulders.
- Lift it off the supports and step back from the rack, setting your feet shoulder-width apart.

MOVE

- Press the weight straight up from your shoulders, tilting your head back so it can clear your chin.
- Once it's past your forehead, bring your head back, and finish the lift with your arms straight and the bar over your ears.
- Lower it along the same path.

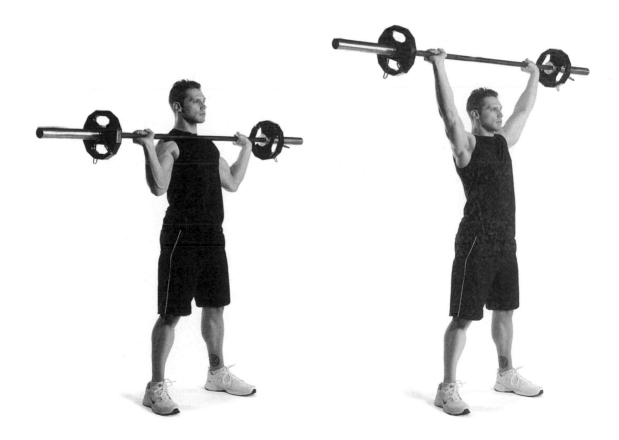

✴ Chin-Up

GET READY

- The Extra Strength program requires you to train with heavier loads and decreasing reps. Alwyn's assumption is that you can do at least 8 chin-ups with your full body weight. That means you need to add weight for sets calling for fewer reps. It's easiest to use a dip belt, a leather or vinyl belt with a chain that allows you to attach weight plates or a dumbbell. (You can get a leather dip belt at performbetter.com for $35 plus shipping.) You can also use a backpack or weighted vest.
- With or without additional weight, grab the chin-up bar with an underhand, shoulder-width grip.

MOVE

- Pull your chest up toward the bar. Your chin should clear the bar by a couple of inches.
- Lower yourself.

VARIATIONS

- As described earlier, you can use band-assisted chin-ups for the higher-rep sets (see the lower left photo on page 161), then use your body weight for intermediate sets, and add weight for the low-rep sets (see the lower right photo on page 161).
- If you can't do chin-ups at all, you can substitute underhand-grip lat pulldowns. Unfortunately, the kneeling version won't work, since you can't really do low-rep, near-maximum-weight sets; the weights will pull you off the floor. So you have to sit on the machine's bench.

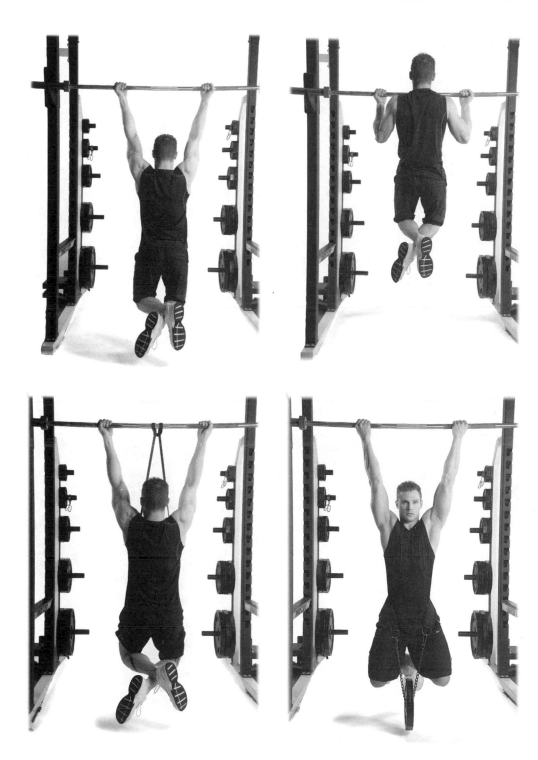

✳ Deadlift

GET READY

- Set up a barbell and roll it to your toes.
- Squat over it with your feet about shoulder-width apart and toes pointed forward.
- Grab it overhand with your arms just outside your legs. (You can use the mixed grip—one hand over the bar, one hand under—for the heaviest sets.)
- Tighten everything up: You want your hips back, knees bent, chest over your thighs, arms straight, shoulders square, eyes forward.

MOVE

- Pull the bar up off the floor, as described earlier.
- Lower the bar to the floor, keeping it as close to your legs as you can. (You might want to wear sweatpants to avoid abrasions.)

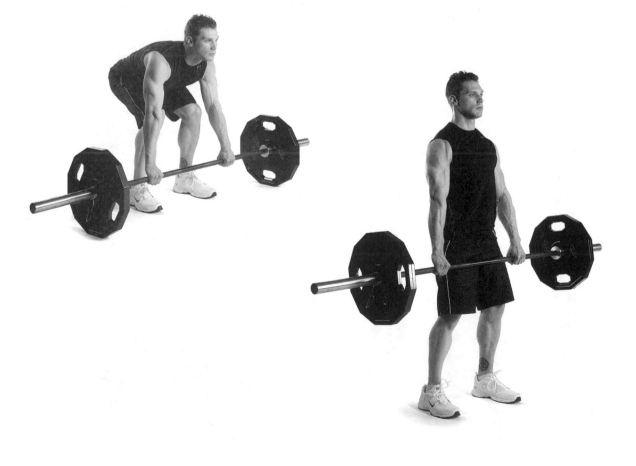

12

Strength: Phase Three

You've probably noticed by now that there's nothing in Alwyn's NROL for Abs program that's "easy." There's no break-in workout, as there was in the original *NROL*. You don't start off with basic exercises, as you did in *NROL for Women*. Some of the exercises in Phase One test your balance and coordination, and the more experienced you are, the tougher the variations you have to choose. In Phase Two the strength exercises are more straightforward, but they're sandwiched by novel and challenging core exercises and metabolic training that tests your fortitude.

Your reward for all that hard work? You're now ready for Phase Three. Which is even harder.

Make no mistake: Hard is good, and harder is better. Unless you were born with the kind of genetics that make it easy to build a lean physique with camera-ready abs, you need a training program that pushes you beyond what you've already done. If your old workouts were going to give you what you want, you'd have it already.

But the workouts have to be the right kind of hard. I get e-mails from readers asking questions about how much they should push themselves, and although there's no specific answer that works for everybody, the general answer is something like this:

You have to get outside your comfort zone. Without someone like Alwyn to design programs for us, we all tend to drift back to the familiar exercises, techniques, and program configurations. They may have been difficult at one point in our development, but now they just reinforce what we already know we can do.

Alwyn's Phase Three workouts have three new elements:

- You'll add one or two power exercises after core training and before the strength program.
- The strength program scraps the traditional system of sets and reps and rest periods. Instead, with each pair of exercises, you'll do as many sets of 6 reps as you can in a 10-minute period. (This system of increasing the volume of work within a defined time period was popularized by Charles Staley, who calls it "escalating density training," or EDT.)
- The metabolic training uses "ladders." You climb the ladder by pushing yourself to do as many reps as you can of the designated exercises, and then you descend the ladder by doing the same workout in reverse order.

As before, you'll start each workout with dynamic mobility. You want to do workouts A and B six to eight times each, and it should take you four to eight weeks to finish Phase Three.

WORKOUT A

Core: Integrated Stabilization			
Exercise	**Sets**	**Reps**	**Rest** (seconds)
1: Turkish get-up	2	5 (each side)	60–90
2: Suitcase deadlift + lateral step-up	2	5 (each side)	60–90
3: Cable anti-rotation reverse lunge with chop	2	8–10 (each side)	60–90
For exercise descriptions, see Chapter 7.			

Power			
Exercise	**Sets**	**Reps**	**Rest** (seconds)
1: Jump shrug			60–90
Week 1	3	5	
Week 2	4	4	
Week 3	5	3	
Week 4*	3	5	
2: Medicine-ball slam (if possible)			60–90
Week 1	3	5	
Week 2	4	4	
Week 3	5	3	
Week 4*	3	5	
*Use same weight as used in week 2.			

How you define a "week" depends on how you plan to proceed through the program. If you expect to train three times a week and complete the program in four weeks, then use "week" literally. Change the sets and reps according to the calendar, no matter how many times you're doing A or B that week.

If you're planning to do A and B 8 times each, then a "week" is two A workouts and two B workouts, no matter how long that is in calendar time.

Strength			
Exercise	**Sets**	**Reps**	**Rest** (seconds)
1a: Split squat, rear foot elevated	AMAP	6 (each leg)	ALAP
1b: Dumbbell plank row	AMAP	6 (each arm)	ALAP
2a: Dumbbell single-leg deadlift with foot on weight plate	AMAP	6 (each leg)	ALAP
2b: Dumbbell chest press on partial bench	AMAP	6 (each arm)	ALAP
AMAP: as many as possible in 10 minutes ALAP: as little as possible			

On all four exercises, use a weight that you'd normally select for 8 reps. Use it on all your sets (unless after the first set you realize it's obviously too heavy or too light). Alternate 1a and 1b for 10 minutes, then for the next 10 minutes alternate 2a and 2b.

Metabolic

In Phase Two, you did burpees for your metabolic training in Workout A, and swings with a dumbbell or kettlebell in Workout B. Now you get to combine them. Start with

10 burpees + 10 swings, then 9 + 9, then 8 + 8, ending with 1 burpee and 1 swing on your final set. Rest as much or as little as you need to between sets.

Each workout, add one rep to your first set. So the second time you do Workout A, you'll do 11 burpees + 11 swings, then continue until you do 1 + 1 for your final set. Thus, by adding a rep to the first set, you're also adding a set to the workout.

WORKOUT B

Core: Integrated Stabilization			
Exercise	Sets	Reps	Rest (seconds)
1: Alligator drag (optional)*	2	10–20 yards	60–90
2: Dumbbell offset farmer's walk (or) Dumbbell offset squat	2	10–20 yards 10–20	60–90
3: Two-Dumbbell offloaded farmer's walk or squat (or) Dumbbell overhead offloaded farmer's walk squat	2	10–20 yards 10–20	60–90

For exercise descriptions, see Chapter 7.

*You can skip this one if you don't have a space to do it at your gym, or if you have social anxiety about doing such an odd-looking exercise in front of others. But it's such a great exercise—and surprisingly fun to do—that I recommend doing it at home if you can't bring yourself to try it at the gym.

Power			
Exercise	Sets	Reps	Rest (seconds)
1: Jump squat			60–90
Week 1	3	5	
Week 2	4	4	
Week 3	5	3	
Week 4*	3	5	
2: Medicine-ball push-pass (if possible)			60–90
Week 1	3	5	
Week 2	4	4	
Week 3	5	3	
Week 4*	3	5	

*Use same weight as used in week 2.

(For explanation of what we mean by a "week," see Workout A.)

Strength			
Exercise	**Sets**	**Reps**	**Rest** (seconds)
1a: Dumbbell reverse lunge with offset loading	AMAP	6 (each leg)	ALAP
1b: Dumbbell incline bench press	AMAP	6	ALAP
2a: Dumbbell one-and-a-quarter squat with heels on weight plate	AMAP	6 (each leg)	ALAP
2b: Close-grip chin-up	AMAP	6 (each arm)	ALAP
AMAP: as many as possible in 10 minutes ALAP: as little as possible Do the strength workout as described for Workout A.			

Metabolic

Do ladders of body-weight squats + push-ups. For your first workout, do 3 squats + 3 push-ups, then 6 + 6, and 9 + 9. Then go down the ladder: 6 + 6, and 3 + 3. That's 27 squats + 27 push-ups.

The next workout, climb a higher ladder: 3 + 3, 6 + 6, 9 + 9, and 12 + 12 at the pinnacle. Then go down the ladder: 9 + 9, 6 + 6, and 3 + 3. That's 48 squats + 48 push-ups.

See how high you can climb. For some of us, the first ladder—27 squats + 27 push-ups—will be all we can handle for a while, since metabolic training follows a fatiguing strength workout, which itself follows uniquely challenging core and power exercises.

POWER EXERCISES

✳ Jump Shrug

GET READY

- Grab a barbell with an overhand, just-beyond-shoulder-width grip, and hold it at arm's length in front of you.
- Stand with your feet shoulder-width apart, hips back, and knees bent, as if you were about to jump. The bar should hang just below your knees.

MOVE

- Jump, straightening your hips and knees and coming all the way off the floor.
- Shrug your shoulders as you come off the ground.

- Cushion your landing by bending your hips and knees as you get into position for the next rep.
- Make progress first by jumping higher and shrugging harder, then by adding more weight.

✳ Jump Squat

GET READY

- Set up a barbell in the squat rack.
- Grab the bar with a wide, overhand grip, and duck your head under it.
- Squeeze your shoulder blades together, forming a shelf with your trapezius muscles to hold the bar.
- Lift the bar off the rack and step back.
- Set your feet shoulder-width apart.

MOVE

- Push your hips back and bend your knees.
- Jump, coming all the way up off the floor.
- Cushion your landing with your hips and knees as you position yourself for the next jump.
- Make progress first by jumping higher, then by adding weight to the bar.

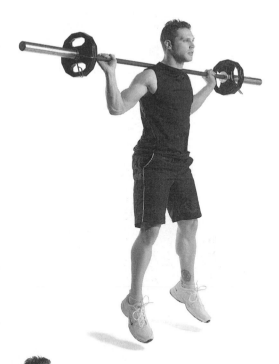

✴ Medicine-Ball Slam

GET READY

- This is a terrific power exercise that almost no one can do in a commercial gym. Lots of gyms have medicine balls, but it's rare to find a club that allows you to throw it to the floor as hard as you can.
- It's also the only exercise in the program in which spinal flexion is a key part of the movement sequence. It's a great movement for competitive athletes in martial arts and any sport that involves throwing.
- If you can do this exercise, you'll need a medicine ball and a floor to throw it against (obviously).
- Stand holding the ball overhead with both hands, your feet shoulder-width apart and your body in an athletic posture, with your knees and hips bent slightly and toes pointed straight ahead.

MOVE

- Slam the ball to the floor with as much force as you can generate.
- Pick it up (if it doesn't bounce back to you) and repeat.
- Make progress first by throwing harder, then by using a heavier ball.

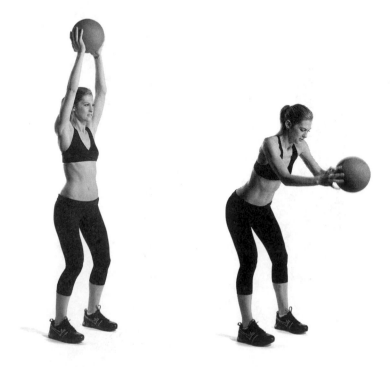

✳ Medicine-Ball Push Pass

GET READY

- This one requires a medicine ball and either a brick or padded wall, or a training partner who'll catch the ball and throw it back.
- Hold the ball with both hands in front of your chest, as if you were going to pass a basketball to a teammate.
- Stand in front of the wall or training partner in an athletic stance.

MOVE

- Step forward with your left leg as you push the ball straight out from your chest with as much force as you can generate.
- Retrieve the ball and repeat, stepping forward with your right leg.
- Make progress first by throwing farther (step back from the wall, or farther away from your partner, and try to hit the same spot), then by using a heavier ball.

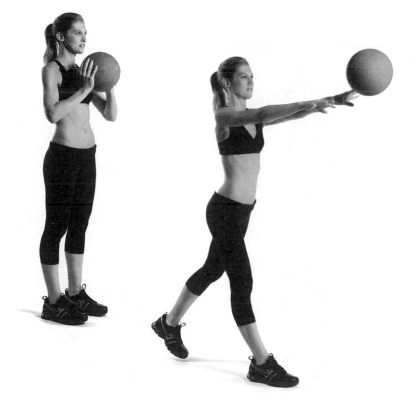

STRENGTH EXERCISES

✳ Split Squat, Rear Foot Elevated

GET READY

- This is the opposite of the front-foot-elevated split squat you did in Phase One. You'll need a low step or box (I recommend no higher than 6 inches) and a pair of dumbbells.
- Hold the dumbbells at arm's length at your sides.
- Start with your dominant foot on the box. Take a long step forward with your nondominant leg, as you would in a lunge.

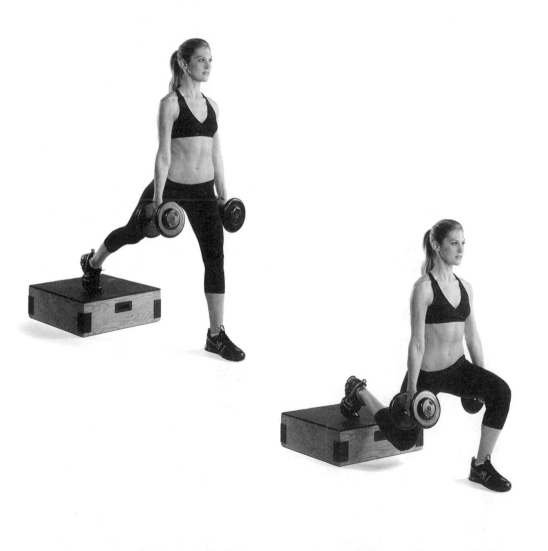

MOVE

- Lower yourself until the thigh of your front leg is parallel to the floor.
- Push back up to the starting position.
- Do 6 reps with your nondominant leg, then switch legs and repeat the set.

CORE CHALLENGE

- Similar to the front-foot-elevated version, it engages all your lower-body muscles, with stabilizing muscles coming into play as the quads, hamstrings, and glutes fatigue.

VARIATIONS

- You can do this with a barbell across the back of your shoulders, holding a weight plate across your chest with both hands, or holding a weight plate directly overhead.
- You can also do an exercise that's usually called the Bulgarian split squat, with the instep of your rear foot resting on a bench. It's harder, and even more of a challenge when you're trying to do the most work possible in a finite block of time.

✳ Dumbbell Plank Row

GET READY

- You'll need a bench and a moderately heavy dumbbell.
- Get into push-up position, with your hands on the bench and your body in a straight line from neck to ankles.
- You want your feet set wide for balance—at least shoulder-width apart until you're familiar with the exercise.
- Reach down and grab the dumbbell with your nondominant hand and hold it at arm's length straight down from your shoulder.

MOVE

- Pull the weight straight up to the side of your abdomen without twisting your legs or torso out of alignment.
- Do 6 reps, then switch to your dominant arm.

CORE CHALLENGE

- If you're having flashbacks to some of the dynamic-stability core exercises you did in Phase Two, you get the idea. This time, core stability is assumed, and you're doing the exercise with a heavy weight to increase muscle strength, size, and endurance.

VARIATION

- You can also do this with a kettlebell.
- The floor version of this exercise, with both hands on dumbbells or kettlebells, is often called a renegade row. It's a terrific exercise for core strength, stability, and endurance, but it's too fatiguing for this part of the program.

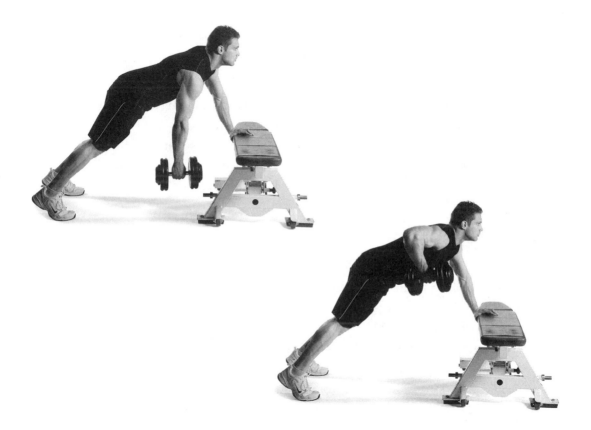

⭑ Dumbbell Single-Leg Deadlift with Foot on Weight Plate

GET READY

- Set a 25- or 45-pound weight plate on the floor, lettered side down.
- Grab a dumbbell that's heavier than the weight you used for the single-leg Romanian deadlift in Phase One.
- Stand on the plate, holding the dumbbell in your right hand at arm's length.
- Without moving your right thigh, bend your right knee 90 degrees, lifting your foot off the floor so your shin is parallel to the floor.

MOVE

- Push your hips back and bend your left knee, lowering the dumbbell as far as you can.
- Rise back to the starting position.
- Do 6 reps, then switch legs and repeat the set.

CORE CHALLENGE

- This exercise, like the wide-grip deadlift from a weight plate in Phase Two, extends the range of motion. But because you're balancing on one leg, with a weight held on your opposite side, you're challenging your core from every direction. You're resisting spinal flexion by keeping your back in the neutral position through a longer range of motion, and you're resisting rotation because of the reduced base of support.

ALTERNATIVES

- You can also do this with two dumbbells, as shown in the photos.

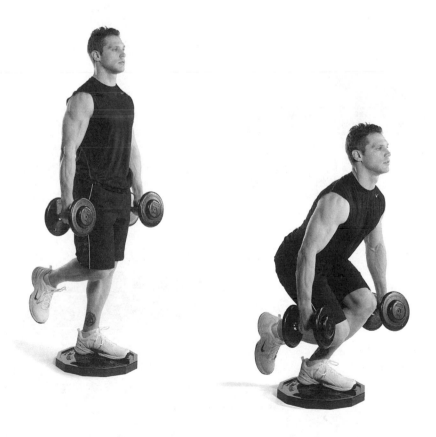

✳ Dumbbell Chest Press on Partial Bench

GET READY

- You'll need a bench and two moderately heavy dumbbells.
- Lay your head and shoulders at one end of a flat bench, with your torso and legs extending from it. You're going to use your body as an extension of the bench.
- Set your feet flat on the floor with your knees bent and your body forming a straight line from your neck to your knees.
- Hold the dumbbells at the edges of your shoulders.

MOVE

- Press the weights straight up, then lower them.

CORE CHALLENGE

- It's similar to the Phase Two chest press, but this time you're pressing two weights at a time, so there's a bit less of an anti-rotation challenge.

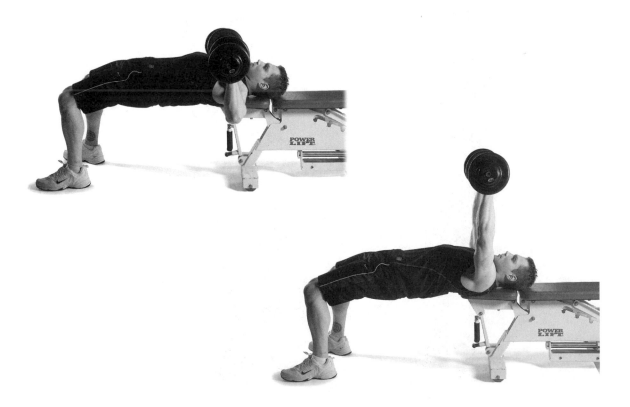

✳ Dumbbell Reverse Lunge with Offset Loading

GET READY

- Grab a moderately heavy dumbbell and hold it next to your right shoulder.
- Stand with your feet hip-width apart.

MOVE

- Step back into a lunge with your left leg, lowering your body until your front thigh is parallel to the floor and your rear knee is close to the floor.
- Push back to the starting position.
- Do 6 reps, then switch the weight to your left hand and repeat the set, stepping back with your right leg.

CORE CHALLENGE

- The offset load challenges your balance and core stability, as you know from similar exercises you've already tried. Don't be afraid to use a heavy weight here; you should be strong enough at this point in the program to load this exercise aggressively.

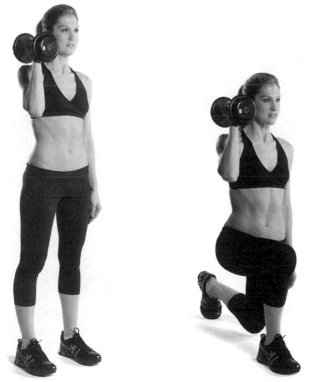

✳ Dumbbell Incline Bench Press

GET READY

- If you've been wondering when you'll get to do a "normal" exercise, this Bud's for you. It's the one exercise in Phase Three that everyone in your gym not only knows how to do, but actually does.
- Set an adjustable bench to an incline—anywhere from 30 to 60 degrees is fine—and grab a pair of dumbbells.
- Lie on your back on the bench with your feet shoulder-width apart and flat on the floor.

MOVE

- Turn to your left and throw the dumbbell in your right hand at the first person you see . . . okay, no, don't do that.
- Press the dumbbells up, lower them, and thank Alwyn for giving you a break.

CORE CHALLENGE

- Because you already know how to do it, you should be able to load up with fairly heavy weights, forcing you to brace your core muscles to strengthen your body's base.

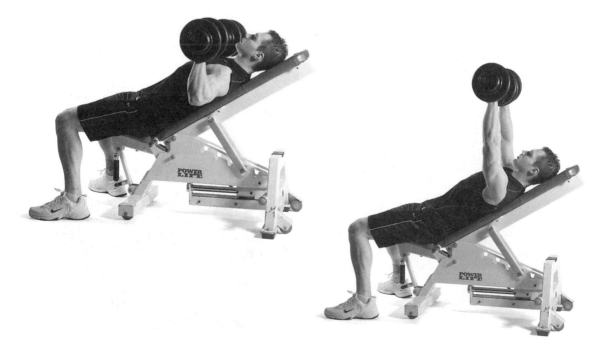

✳ Dumbbell One-And-A-Quarter Squat with Heels on Weight Plates

GET READY

- Now that you've had your fun with a traditional exercise, we're back to the unusual.
- Set a pair of weight plates on the floor—5- or 10-pounders will do.
- Grab a pair of dumbbells and hold one at your left shoulder, with the other at your right side.
- Place your heels on the weight plates with your feet shoulder-width apart and toes pointed forward or angled out slightly.

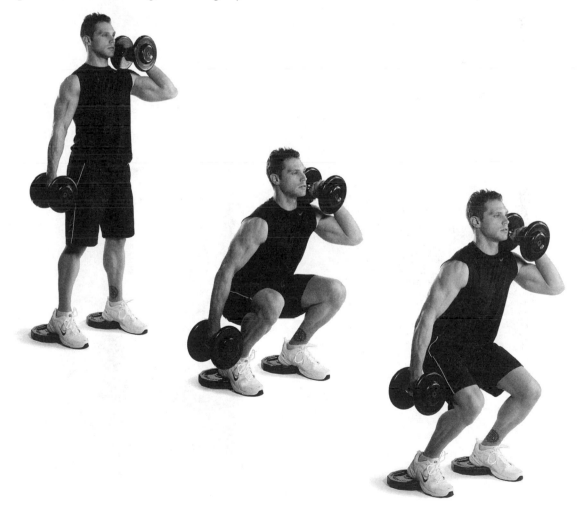

MOVE

- Push your hips back and squat down until your thighs are parallel to the floor.
- Rise a quarter of the way back to the starting position.
- Lower yourself again.
- Rise to the starting position. That's one repetition.
- Do 6 reps, put the weights down, and go on to the next exercise. Switch the weights for the next set, so you're holding them at your right shoulder and left side.

CORE CHALLENGE

- You're getting it from all directions. It's a bit easier to hold your spine in the neutral position with your heels raised, but much harder to prevent rotation with the weights at two different heights.

✳ Close-Grip Chin-Up

GET READY

- Grab the chin-up bar with an underhand grip that's less than shoulder width.
- Hang from the bar with your arms straight, knees bent, and ankles crossed behind you.

MOVE

- Pull your chest up toward the bar. Your chin should clear the bar by a couple of inches.

CORE CHALLENGE

- Moving your hands closer together makes the exercise a little easier, since you're getting help from your biceps, along with your upper-torso muscles. (One of the most unexpected things you learn when you read about exercise science is

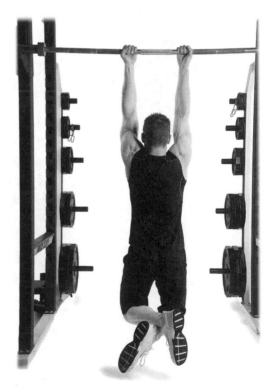

that the chest muscles assist on close-grip pull-ups and chin-ups.) But since you'll be doing a lot more chin-ups than you did with previous versions, the net effect is more work for all your muscles.

VARIATIONS

- Most of us won't be able to do many sets of 6 chin-ups, even with the close grip. So your goal here is to increase the total number of chin-ups you can do in 10 minutes every time you do the workout, even if the last few sets are just 1 or 2 reps. As long as you can do 3 or 4 reps in the first couple of sets, it's better to do chin-ups than lat pulldowns.

- You can also do the band-assisted chin-up, shown on page 161, lower left, or a combination of the two. Start with regular chin-ups, then switch to band-assisted as you get tired.

- As a last resort, you can do kneeling close-grip lat pulldowns, or neutral-grip pulldowns using the triangle-shaped handle. It's still a good exercise, even if it's not the best one.

PART 4

ABS, LOST AND FOUND

The Anti-Abs Conspiracy

EACH PERSON READING this book is probably heavier than he or she would have been a generation ago. We're so used to having a bigger population that we don't think about it much. But our increased heft really is a generational leap forward. The average woman is nineteen pounds heavier than her counterpart from the late 1970s, while the average man has been upsized by seventeen pounds.

The simple explanation is that we eat more and exercise less than we used to. It's easy enough to agree with the first half of the statement. In 1970, there were 2,172 calories of food available in the United States per person per day, adjusted for waste. By 2007, there were 2,775 calories available—a 28 percent increase. About 300 of those extra calories came from added fats (a whopping 73 percent increase), with about 200 from grains (a 45 percent bump), and another 57 from added sugars (up 14 percent).

So I don't think anybody disputes the argument that we eat a lot more food than our parents or grandparents did. The question is, why? Sure, food is cheaper, relative to our paychecks. And yes, there's more of it wherever we turn than there used to be. But I don't eat based on what I can afford, or on what I can see when I look around. I eat because I'm hungry. I assume you do too.

I'm left with two potential answers to the question: Either the food supply has changed, meaning we need more food to feel satisfied than we did a generation ago, or we're hungrier than we used to be, for reasons that have nothing to do with our food.

Alas, both are almost certainly true.

I'll address our diabolically reengineered food supply in Chapter 14. For now, let's look at some of the reasons why we're hungrier than we used to be.

NEW RULE #10 • You can't out-exercise a hunger-inducing lifestyle.

If we exercise less today than we used to, as some in the food industry desperately want us to believe, virtually everyone should lose weight the minute they start a fitness program. But that's not what happens.

I'll give you one example: In a 2008 study published in the *International Journal of Obesity*, thirty-five sedentary, overweight men and women took part in a twelve-week exercise program. Average weight loss in the group was about eight pounds. *Individual* results, however, ranged from a loss of thirty-two pounds to a gain of almost four pounds. How much would you hate the world if you exercised five days a week for three months and ended up *gaining* weight?

I'm not saying exercise doesn't help with weight and fat control. It does. But, as an isolated intervention, it clearly doesn't work for everybody who hits the gym or laces up running shoes. And even if it did offer a linear path to weight loss, you could never exercise enough to make up for the factors that caused you to gain too much weight in the first place.

NEW RULE #11 • Your computer is the enemy of your abs.

Back in 1990, researchers at the University of Washington School of Medicine ran a clever experiment: They tested the increase in stress experienced by employees of their university who were in charge of processing grant proposals. The flow of proposals into the Grant and Contract Services office was entirely predictable; there were three periods each year when they were swamped, and other times when the workload was comparatively light. Two of the crunch-time periods served as examples of how the employees reacted to stress, while a low-workload period was used as the "control" setting.

The researchers were most concerned with changes in cholesterol levels during periods of stress, with the idea that this was the mechanism by which stress led to heart disease. Assuming cholesterol would rise, they had to identify what fueled the increase. That's why they measured calorie intake during high- and low-stress periods. Sure enough, employees ate about 240 more calories a day when stressed.

The results were interesting, sure, but the experiment had some limitations. First, because the employees were doing vital work under deadline pressure, the researchers couldn't control the tasks they actually performed. Second, their blood tests focused on cholesterol, instead of looking at hormones that are directly linked to stress, like cortisol. Third, the participants recorded their food consumption in diaries, a notoriously inaccurate way to track calories. (People chronically underreport how much they eat, either because they forget or because they don't want to say.)

Eighteen years later, obesity researchers at Laval University in Quebec tackled the

Brain Candy

When I use the term "blood sugar," I'm talking about glucose, which is the form of readily available carbohydrate energy that circulates throughout your body. (It's stored in your muscles and liver in a slightly different form, called glycogen.) Blood sugar is one of your body's simplest and most dependable regulators of hunger. If everything's working correctly, you should get hungry when it drops, and stop being hungry when it rises.

Throughout the day, your body relies on fat for most of its energy needs. A small amount of fat circulates in your blood, with an even smaller amount stored within your muscles. Your meals provide your body with plenty of new fat throughout the day, which it can use for energy. And if you need more—that is, if you're in a state of *negative energy balance*, meaning you're using more energy than you're taking in—your body can find abundant amounts within your fat cells.

We tend to think of our muscles as our body's major drivers of fuel consumption, but it's actually the brain that jacks up the cost of being human. It represents just 2 percent of your body's weight, but uses 20 percent of its energy. While your muscles fuel themselves with a mixture of fat and blood sugar, your brain runs on pure glucose. (This despite the fact it's made mostly of fat.)

Of course your body can turn fat into glucose and your brain will operate just fine. You can follow a very-low-carbohydrate diet with no fear of turning into a drooling moron. So when we talk about how stressful, deadline-driven, brain-draining work makes your body think it needs more fuel, we don't mean you're driven to eat more sugar. Maybe you are, maybe you aren't. The key finding of the studies discussed in this chapter is that you're driven to eat more food because of knowledge work, not that you're seeking out any particular type of food.

same questions, but with better controls. They measured the metabolism and stress responses of fourteen student volunteers under three conditions: sitting in a comfy chair and doing nothing; reading an assigned text and then writing a 350-word report on it; or doing a challenging assignment on a computer with potential distractions. Each condition lasted forty-five minutes.

Then they measured how much food the volunteers ate from a buffet after each part of the experiment.

The amount of calories burned by the volunteers was nearly identical during each test, as you'd expect. Since there wasn't any physical exertion involved, it only took a few more calories to do the "knowledge-based work" than it had to relax in a chair.

However, the food consumption afterward was remarkably different. The volunteers ate an average of 203 calories more after the reading-and-writing test, compared with the part of the experiment where they sat in chairs and did nothing. And after they had to work on a computer for forty-five minutes, they ate 253 more calories. The more *perceived* effort it took to complete an intellectual task, the more the subjects' blood-sugar levels fluctuated, and the hungrier they were afterward.

NEW RULE #12 • TV and video games are almost as bad as your computer.

Or they might be worse. We don't know yet, although the preliminary evidence is disturbing. A team of Australian researchers found that adults who watched the most TV—more than 2.57 hours a day for the men, 2.14 hours a day for the women—had the largest waist circumference. That's just one of the markers of metabolic mayhem the study measured, but it's obviously the one we're most concerned with in a book that has "abs" in the title.

Here's the kicker: The four thousand people in this study weren't slugs. They all reported at least two and a half hours a week of "moderate- to vigorous-intensity physical activity." That's a decent amount of exercise. And yet the more time they spent in front of the TV, the more belly fat they accumulated.

The previous section showed that knowledge-based work causes blood-sugar fluctuations, which in turn stimulate appetite. Exercise has been shown to help minimize those fluctuations. So, in theory, a good workout program can mitigate the damage to your waistline caused by computer work. But with TV, the only way to limit the damage is to limit the amount of time you spend in front of it.

It's an open question whether video games are more like knowledge work or more like watching TV, in terms of the metabolic toll on your body. One study, published in 2009 in the *American Journal of Preventive Medicine*, found that adult game players are heavier than non-players and tend to have worse physical and mental health.

Does one cause the other, or do people who're fatter and more depressed just spend more of their time playing video games? It's too early to say. The big point I'm trying to make here is that TV and video games, at worst, are part of an electronic army marching from virtual Mordor to wage war on your body composition. At best they're merely correlated with that battle for control of your waistline. Either way, they represent a lifestyle choice that hinders your pursuit of a leaner physique.

NEW RULE #13 • You can sleep your way to a better body . . . or not sleep your way to a bigger belly.

Consider this statement from a paper by two University of Chicago researchers: "In recent years, sleep curtailment has become a hallmark of modern society, with both children and adults having shorter bedtimes than a few decades ago. This trend for shorter sleep duration has developed over the same time period as the dramatic increase in the prevalence of obesity."

You almost never hear the issue framed in such stark terms. And, indeed, I don't think anyone puts *all* the blame for the rise in body weight on a lack of sleep. But bad sleep habits do play a part.

Let's start with cortisol, the stress hormone. Normally, as you approach bedtime, your cortisol level falls rapidly. At the same time, a hormone called leptin rises. Leptin, in a healthy body, is a powerful appetite suppressor. Rising leptin and falling cortisol make for an ideal sleep environment. Low hunger, low stress—you should sleep like a baby. (The kind of baby who sleeps through the night, I mean. My wife and I have experience with both kinds.)

But with chronic sleep loss, the two hormones fall out of synch. Leptin peaks before bedtime, then falls just when it should be rising. Cortisol doesn't fall as fast as it should. The result is that you're stressed and hungry—a horrible combination any time of day, but especially damaging just when you're trying to fall asleep.

It's even worse when you wake up in the morning. In conditions of chronic sleep debt, you have problems with another hormone: insulin. You probably know that insulin is a storage hormone; it shuttles nutrients from your bloodstream to the tissues where they're needed. When you eat after a workout, for example, insulin pushes glucose into your muscles to replace the fuel that powered your training, along with protein to repair them and build new muscle tissue.

You need insulin to function optimally in the morning, because that's when cortisol is at its highest point of the day, and leptin is at its lowest. The cortisol-induced stress helps you wake up, and the leptin-induced hunger ensures that you fill your stomach following so many hours without food. You have fewer inhibitions with that high-cortisol, low-leptin combo special (this is probably why doughnuts became a staple of America's breakfast buffet), and whatever you eat is soon going to hit your bloodstream like a glucose tsunami.

Two things need to happen:

- Your body has to recognize that all these nutrients are suddenly available.
- Insulin must work quickly and efficiently to move the sugar and fat out of your blood.

If both those mechanisms are functioning properly, as they should following a full night's sleep, you'll feel satiated and won't be hungry again for hours. If they aren't, you probably won't.

One study from the University of Chicago research team found that after just two days of restricted sleep, hunger shot up 24 percent overall. But hunger for high-carbohydrate food increased 32 percent.

That explains why sleep loss makes you fatter. Combine truncated sleep routines with the ravages of stressful knowledge work, followed by hours unwinding in front of the TV, and you have a formula that could keep your abs hidden for your entire adult life.

You Gotta Move

The problems I just described have self-evident solutions:

1. Don't let your computer or TV determine your activity level.
2. Learn where the "off" switches are on your laptop and cell phone, and use them.
3. Go to sleep at the same time every night. If you're going to allow an exception, make it something that's really worth staying up for. (For me, it's the seventh game of the World Series . . . but only if my team is playing.)

Specifically, one of the best and simplest strategies is to move more, and move more often. One study reported this: "On average, each 10 percent increase in sedentary time was associated with a 3.1-centimeter larger waist circumference." That's about 1.25 inches. The same researchers found that taking more breaks—getting up off your chair and walking around, no matter how far or fast you walk—was linked to smaller waist sizes. Of the 168 middle-aged subjects they studied, the waist measurements of the ones who got up most often were more than two inches smaller than those who got up the least.

People like us—men and women who're willing to go to the gym two or three times a week and work hard once we get there—don't think of ourselves as sedentary. But many of us have jobs that force us to sit for extended lengths of time, and sitting is a self-perpetuating activity. The less we move, the more weight we gain. The more weight we gain, the less we move.

The simple act of standing up forces muscles to contract, particularly those in your glutes and thighs. It allows you to straighten out the hip-flexor muscles that tend to get shorter and weaker with extended sitting. And if you pull your shoulders back when you stand, you also stretch out the pectoralis minor, a chest muscle that, like the hip flexors, tends to adaptively shorten with extended hunching over a keyboard.

The Evening Ramble

As I mentioned in Chapter 8, the NROL for Abs program includes some sort of physical activity every day of the week, including the days you do Alwyn's workouts. It could be as simple and informal as an evening walk, jog, or bike ride, or as regimented as a yoga class or team sport. It's up to you. It just needs to fulfill three requirements:

1. You're up and moving.
2. You aren't in front of a TV or computer, or answering calls on your cell phone.
3. It involves something you enjoy.

The goal isn't to burn a significant number of calories, although it's fine if you do. It's to burn *some* energy while getting you away from the things that affect your appetite, mood, and activity level in a bad way—your TV, computer, and cell phone. The calories you use in that evening walk won't have a huge impact on your waistline, but they aren't entirely negligible. Researchers from the Mayo Clinic have suggested that one aspect of modern life—the fact that hardly any of us walk to work anymore—by itself can account for almost all the surplus calories needed to become obese over time.

There are better and worse ways to get your daily exercise. Here's a good one I wouldn't have thought of: When I saw my brother-in-law last Christmas, he looked quite a bit leaner than he had the previous winter. I asked what had changed. Nothing, he said, except that he spent more time walking his two dogs. He lives in the southwest U.S., so the weather rarely keeps him from getting his evening walk.

Indeed, preliminary research from the University of Missouri College of Veterinary Medicine suggests that people who walk dogs get more and better exercise than people who walk with their fellow humans. That's because humans will slow each other down or talk themselves out of walking altogether, whereas dogs won't argue at all.

Create Your Own Sleeper Cell

It's easy enough for someone like me to say, "Sleep more." Actually pulling it off is quite a bit harder. For some of us, the problem is a work or class schedule that runs counter to our natural circadian rhythm. Take me, for example: I'm a morning person who always made it to my eight a.m. classes in college. (I was paying my own way, and I figured that skipping a class I'd paid to attend was tantamount to running a business but not requiring my employees to show up for work.) But as an adult, when I have to attend a seminar or lecture at night, I struggle to retain the information. I'm an A student before lunch and a C-minus student after dinner.

My heart goes out to the "night people" whose jobs require them to be alert and productive early in the morning. And the people who have to do shift work are in circadian hell; whether they're early or late risers by nature, no one is supposed to work from midnight to eight a.m., and then sleep during the day.

Having children is a sneaky sleep thief, especially for women. Once a new mother trains herself to wake up whenever the infant cries, it's difficult to relearn how to sleep through the night.

So how do you sleep better? Some tips from a variety of sources:

1. Don't try to recover lost sleep by napping or changing your normal sleep schedule. You'll just compound the problem.
2. Caffeine and alcohol can throw off your normal cycle of alertness followed by sleepiness. If you have trouble falling asleep and suspect that caffeine is to blame, give yourself arbitrary cutoff times—no coffee or tea after four p.m., for example.

As for alcohol, you just have to pick the moments when it's worthwhile to indulge, and balance those with evenings when you drink less than you otherwise would.

3. Try lowering the temperature of your bedroom. A cooler room helps your body reduce its core temperature, which is necessary for deep sleep.

4. The information on exercise and sleep is all over the place. Most sources seem to agree that exercise during the day helps you sleep better at night. (If nothing else, it makes your body more tired.) But exercising in the evening can have either effect—leaving you too stimulated to fall asleep at your normal time, or so tired you fall asleep before your head hits the pillow.

5. Playing or coaching sports in the evening always keeps me up later than usual. For me, the excitement of competition takes hours to wear off, whereas simple exercise—an evening walk or bike ride—has no effect on my sleep.

6. As I said earlier, you need to find the "off" switch on your computer and cell phone. I can't offer specific data on this, but in my own experience, the earlier I shut off the electronics in the evening, the easier it is to fall asleep that night.

7. Lots of people fall asleep in front of the TV, which is something I've never been able to pull off. If I happen to fall asleep with the TV on—when I'm trying to stay up late to watch a ball game, for example—the sound and the light of the TV inevitably wake me up a short time later. As soon as I turn off the TV, I'm wide awake, and stay that way for hours. My advice is to turn the TV off before bedtime.

8. Noise and light have highly personal effects on sleep quality. I can't sleep without silence and darkness, but you might need some background noise and ambient light.

9. Avoid using a loud alarm to wake up in the morning. The acute stress it causes will affect your mood in the morning, and fear of the alarm will have long-term consequences. You'll have more anxiety at night, thinking about how much you hate the sound of the alarm in the morning, and you'll wake up each subsequent morning feeling as if you've been robbed of valuable sleep.

10. I'm not much of a supplement pusher. But my teen- and tweenage kids take melatonin at night, and say it helps them sleep. I sometimes take an antihistamine at bedtime when I'm stuffed up during allergy season, and it always helps. I try to minimize it, though, since antihistamines are known to cause "rebound congestion"—creating the problem they're designed to alleviate.

The Problem
with Processing

My FATHER WAS an exceptionally fat individual. At a time when virtually no white-collar, middle-class men got a lick of exercise, and all the men in our neighborhood achieved a saggy-jowled kind of squishiness as a group signifier, my dad was *still* exceptionally fat. Malcolm Gladwell would've considered him an outlier.

Dad, to his credit, worked hard to achieve his girth. You had to back then. Family dinners were mostly the old-fashioned meat and potatoes. Even if the meat came from the fattiest cuts and the potatoes were soaked in butter and sour cream, there was only so much of it anyone could eat at one sitting. What he couldn't achieve with volume, he made up for with frequency, supplementing his three squares with daily fast food. But even fast food in the sixties and seventies wasn't the ticket to fat city it later became. Portion sizes were a fraction of what they are now.

If you took my forty-five-year-old father from 1970 and dropped him in among a group of demographically similar men today, he wouldn't be an outlier at all. He'd probably look softer and fleshier (my totally unscientific observation is that extremely overweight men today seem wider, rounder, and more filled-out than the ones I saw growing up), but you wouldn't pick him out of a crowd.

To me personally, this is as good a sign as any that the current food supply is dramatically different from the one many of us grew up with in the sixties and seventies. What my dad achieved through a pure desire to overeat can be surpassed today without any effort at all. You can get more food in less time, with less hassle and for less money (relative to the price of everything else) than you could thirty years ago. You can eat it faster, and your body probably will be satiated for a shorter interval before you get hungry again.

The problem of an increasingly processed food supply has led many fitness enthusiasts to embrace "clean eating," a concept that means something slightly different to everyone who tries it.

But before I get into the benefits and shortcomings of eating clean, I want to take a closer look at the reason we're talking about clean eating in the first place.

NEW RULE #14 • "Convenience" food is designed for one reason: to make you eat more convenience food.

I like to think I'm a reality-based adult. For example, I believe most individuals will instinctively act in their own self-interest most of the time. The actions of governments, businesses, and social organizations, in theory, should resemble those of individuals. Since it's not in the interest of organizations or individuals to kill off their customers and constituents, society-wide self-interest should provide built-in regulating mechanisms.

But as we all know, self-interest unmoored from moral, legal, or civic constraints will produce one disaster after another. The tobacco industry is the perfect example. It manipulated products to make them more addictive, marketed the products to people who were too young to purchase them legally, and fought any effort to regulate its products or portray them as hazardous to anyone's health.

Which brings me to the food industry. I really had no idea how far restaurants and processed-food manufacturers had gone down the path carved by the tobacco industry until I read *The End of Overeating* by David A. Kessler, M.D., a former commissioner of the U.S. Food and Drug Administration.

Here's the basic idea: The human appetite is aroused by palatable foods. If you make foods more palatable, people will eat more of them, even if those people aren't hungry, or if they've already eaten enough to satisfy their biological needs. The food industry figured out that sugar, fat, and salt are the three categories of nutrients that make food so appetizing it's hard to stop eating once you start. Therefore, if you're in the business of packaging and selling food products, and have a vested interest in getting people to buy and consume more of your products, you add and then manipulate sugar, fat, and salt until you've made those products irresistible. Even meat products served in restaurants are manipulated to require less chewing, which allows us to eat faster and thus eat more before our stomach has a chance to send satiety signals to our brain.

Then you use all the tricks of marketing to associate the products with good times and social status: the Super Bowl party shown in the commercial is at *your* house, with all *your* young and attractive friends watching the game in *your* living room, on *your* flat-screen TV, while coincidentally eating the chips and dip you've purchased. The marketers know this cascade of stimuli will wear down people until they're conditioned to overeat even in the absence of their young and attractive friends.

Entire books have been written to make the argument that human body weight (and, by extension, body composition) is genetically determined. The fanciful idea is that people are fatter now because we finally have enough cheap and readily available food to allow *Homo sapiens* to achieve our full potential for corpulence.

The truth is different: We're fatter because we eat too much *now*, not because our ancestors ate too little then. It's impossible to say exactly why people eat more, but the

Downsizing Satan

Back in 2002, I worked with a team of writers and editors to produce a book called *The Men's Health Belly-Off Program*. The book never got any traction—I think we gave away more copies than we sold—but it presented at least one idea that probably was novel at that time in the mainstream media. My colleagues and I wrote about a sinister new interloper in the food chain: high-fructose corn syrup, or HFCS.

I repeated the charge in the original *NROL*, which came out in 2006, referring to HFCS as an "evil food" and "metabolic nightmare." By the time we wrote *NROL for Women*, published in 2008, I was hedging my bets, calling HFCS "cheaper and potentially worse for you than traditional sweeteners made from sugarcane."

I'll stand behind "cheaper," and a cheaper sweetener is one that allows larger portion sizes, which in turn lead to larger belly sizes. But I'm calling myself out on the rest. In truth, HFCS is just another sugar. Table sugar—sucrose—is about 50 percent fructose and 50 percent glucose. Fructose is a sugar found in fruits, vegetables, and nuts. You already know what glucose is; in nature, it's found wherever you'll find fructose. HFCS is basically the same thing, only with a slightly higher amount of fructose, typically 55 percent instead of 50. As the poet said, whoop-de-doo.

changes in the food supply, making the things we eat both tastier and less satiating, almost certainly have a lot to do with it.

NEW RULE #15 • Processed food makes you stupid and depressed.

A team of researchers at University College London studied a middle-aged population of office workers in the UK. They found that the ones who ate the most processed food had the highest rates of depression. The category includes refined grains, processed meat, sweetened desserts, fried food, and high-fat dairy products.

Even after they adjusted for all the potential confounders—including age, education, and lifestyle factors like smoking and exercise—those who ate the most processed food were 58 percent more likely to suffer from depression, compared to those who ate the least.

That same research team also found a strong association between processed food and cognitive deficits associated with dementia. Compared to those who ate the least processed food, those who ate the most were worse at tests that measured vocabulary and reasoning. Interestingly, though, the links between diet and dementia got a lot weaker when the researchers adjusted for the amount of education their subjects had attained. People with less education are more likely to eat processed food, and people with more education are less likely to suffer from dementia no matter what they eat.

Still, there are obvious patterns here. The numbers all run in one direction: People who eat the most processed food have more depression and less cognitive ability. Those who eat the most whole food have the least depression and the most brainpower in old age.

NEW RULE #16 • All that said, calories still matter more than anything else.

Let's pretend we're setting up a scientific experiment. For the next six months, a pair of identical twins, Tweedledee and Tweedledum, will eat the exact same volume of food, with the same number of meals, consumed at the same time. Their ratios of protein, carbs, and fat will be identical. They'll get the same amount of fiber, and sufficient amounts of vitamins and minerals. They'll do the same training program.

The only difference is that Tweedledee will get all of his or her food from "clean" sources—whole foods like fruits, vegetables, eggs, fish, meat, dairy, and poultry. If you want to make it *really* clean, we can say all the food is certified organic and free-range, and personally supervised from zygote to harvest by a Norwegian bachelor farmer with dual Ph.D.'s in ethics and sustainable ecology. He reads poetry to the tomatoes, teaches conflict resolution to the bulls, and convinces the roosters to use their indoor voice.

Tweedledum gets his or her meals delivered from local fast-food joints, and takes vitamin, mineral, and fiber supplements to make up for the deficiencies of the burgers and fries.

If you ask which one would be happier and healthier a year or ten years down the road, assuming they maintain these extreme diets, of course I'd vote for the one eating the pesticide-free carrots and eggs that come from chickens with high self-esteem. But if you ask which one will gain more muscle or lose more fat during the six-month experiment, my honest guess is that it would be a tie.

Weight control still comes down to calories. Eat more than you burn off, and you gain weight. Burn off more than you take in, and you lose fat. You should be able to achieve any fitness- or physique-related goal you want with any diet you choose, so long as you control the amount you eat, get enough protein, and avoid nutritional deficiencies.

What We Need from Our Food

The key word in the previous sentence: *control.*

We all hear about people who can eat anything they want and stay lean, thanks to intense training programs or freakish metabolic rates. And we hear about people who meticulously plan each meal but gain weight if the wind blows a stray carpet fiber into their bowl of organic lentils. But most of us live between those two extremes. For us, the best diet is the one that gives us the most functional value, the most nutritional value, and the greatest satiety, with the least amount of inconvenience.

Here's how I define those categories:

Functional value: Function starts with enough calories to reach your goal, whether you're trying to gain something, lose something, or maintain what you currently have. You want your food to provide enough energy to perform your workouts at a high level, and to recover from them afterward. You want enough protein to build muscle, and enough fiber to ensure regularity. And, although this is amorphous and highly individual, you also want to feel good, which means your diet should include the foods that elevate your mood and avoid the ones that make you feel sad, bloated, or sluggish.

Nutritional value: I don't know if you can "feel" nutritional value, but it's something we all worry about, with good reason. So even if you don't notice any functional difference, you probably feel guilty on the days you don't eat your fruits and vegetables. You know you're supposed to eat a multicolored variety of plants so you get a multicolored variety of health benefits. All those vitamins, minerals, and hard-to-pronounce micronutrients have been linked to longer lives and less risk of disease, and you want a ticket on that train before it leaves the station.

Satiety: There's no one standard for satiety, although I think most of us expect a substantial meal to tide us over for at least four hours. A good snack should reduce hunger pangs for the next two hours. Whatever the timetable, we don't want to feel hungry between meals. And when we get to the end of the day, we don't want to feel as if we've been deprived of anything.

Convenience: I work at home, so it's theoretically possible for me to plan, shop for, and prepare every bite I eat without ever touching anything that comes in a box, bag, or can. And yet I eat Kashi Go Lean cereal every morning for breakfast, I snack on a protein bar from time to time, and the meats and produce my wife prepares for dinner come from the same grocery aisles everyone else uses. (The leftovers provide the next day's lunch, in case you were wondering.)

Why don't I cook an omelet or prepare steel-cut oats for breakfast? Because it's inconvenient. Why aren't my wife and I trolling the farmers' markets for locally grown, certified-organic food? Same answer.

The produce we eat undoubtedly comes laced with pesticides, while the meat, eggs, and dairy products contain hormones and antibiotics. Then you add the chemicals that leach into food from plastic or metal containers, and you subtract the nutrients that might be lost when "fresh" produce is flown in from the other side of the world so we can enjoy raspberries in January. And yet, for all its limitations and potential risks, this is my version of "clean" eating, or as close as I'm ever going to get. If it means I die at 90 instead of 91.5, I'll just have to live with that. Or not live. Whichever.

My diet follows most of the advice and recommendations I'll make in the next few chapters. Other than the cereal for breakfast and protein bars for snacks, I eat very few prepared or packaged meals. We don't eat out much, and when we do, it's usually at a sit-down restaurant, with food that (we hope) is prepared to order. Our main goal

How a Fitness Buff Thinks About Food

In *The Body Fat Solution*, bodybuilder and author Tom Venuto notes that someone who's focused on performance and physique goals will view food in four completely utilitarian ways:

1. Food is building material.

When a gym rat drinks a protein shake before, during, and/or after a workout, he's thinking about that protein going directly to his muscles. Of course it doesn't really work that way—a typical protein shake might have 40 grams of protein, but if an experienced lifter gains a few grams of actual muscle tissue a week, he's doing extremely well. Still, thinking about food as *something that becomes a permanent part of your body* certainly helps you make better choices.

2. Food is fuel.

Same thought, only this time your focus is on generating energy for your workouts, rather than making permanent additions to your physical being.

3. Food is nourishment.

Aside from tissue-building and activity-fueling, most of us worry about whether we're getting what we need for long-term health. If you think about how a doughnut or an order of French fries might affect your chance of getting heart disease or cancer, you don't eat those foods. We understand that a few hundred calories of greasy guilt here and there, in the context of a lifetime that includes millions of total calories, will have little impact. But thinking about your future health does make that salad a lot more appetizing.

4. Food stokes the metabolic fire.

I'll cover meals and metabolism in more detail in Chapter 15. For now, I'll just note that people who read fitness magazines and buy workout books probably understand that it takes calories to process calories. That's why eating increases your metabolic rate. Those who think of food only in terms of storage—"this sandwich will go straight to my waistline"—will be afraid to eat. Those who see food as an important driver of their metabolism, which is key to getting and staying lean, will have a healthier attitude toward their meals.

is to eat as little processed food as possible, which means that most of our meals are built around food that's as close to its natural state as we can manage.

Still, I understand that my version of a "clean" diet might be shockingly unclean by your standards. My goal isn't to bring you down to my level if you're already doing better. All the nutrition information in this book is designed to help you make the best choices for your needs and your circumstances.

Nutrition Made Simple . . . Well, *Kind of Simple*

HERE'S WHAT YOU NEED to survive, assuming an adequate supply of oxygen:

1. Water
2. Food

That's it. You can go a few days without any water at all, and several weeks without food. But as long as you aren't completely dehydrated and you have some source of energy that prevents your body from devouring its own tissues, you can keep on living for an indeterminate length of time—weeks, months, even years.

Now, here's what you need to thrive as a healthy, active adult, free of the major diseases linked to nutritional deprivation:

1. Water

Your muscles are about 75 percent water, as is as much as two-thirds of your body weight. Even your bones are 22 percent H_2O. Your brain? Three-quarters liquid. On average, you probably need three quarts of fluids a day to stay fully hydrated; about a half quart will come from your food. (Bread, for example, is 35 percent water; fruits and vegetables might be as much as 90 percent.) Drinking more than that might increase your metabolism a bit, or perhaps help you feel fuller so you eat less at meals. My own hunch is that excess fluids help with weight control because they send you to the bathroom more often. That means you get up and move around more throughout the day.

2. Food

Although the math gets complicated, I'll pull some numbers out of the air and guess that an average 180-pound man will lose weight if he eats fewer than 1,800 calories a day, and a 140-pound woman will lose weight on fewer than 1,400. Everything ·affects these numbers. For starters: height and weight, age, physical activity, body composition, meal patterns, and food choices.

3. Protein

If most of your body is water, what's the rest? Protein, mainly. Protein makes up about 20 percent of your muscles, heart, liver, and glands, and 10 percent of your brain. Most of your hormones, antibodies, and enzymes—the chemicals that make life possible—are made of protein. And although we think of our bones as hardened minerals like calcium, the outer part is actually collagen, a critical protein that also forms tendons and ligaments, and strengthens blood vessels.

Your body is constantly breaking down and rebuilding the protein in its tissues, especially in your muscles after a workout. Logically, you'd assume you need a lot of protein. The truth is that you need relatively little protein to survive, but your body will thrive on more.

4. Fat

As with protein, you can survive on relatively small amounts; your body mainly needs fat for energy, either to use immediately or store in your fat cells. Without any you wouldn't be able to absorb four vitamins (A, D, E, and K), and you'd suffer lower production of two crucial hormones: testosterone and estrogen. In one yearlong study, a diet that was only modestly low in fat—about 20 percent of total calories—lowered estrogen by 7.5 percent. (And that's assuming the women in the study complied with its guidelines, which is unlikely over twelve months.)

5. Vitamins and minerals

We know humans are susceptible to health problems related to nutritional deficiencies, among them scurvy (vitamin C), rickets (vitamin D), osteoporosis (calcium), beriberi (vitamin B1), and anemia (iron), for starters. All of these can be avoided with a diet that includes a variety of foods. You can get your vitamin C from fruits and vegetables, vitamin D and calcium from dairy foods, iron from meat or beans, and B vitamins from meat and fortified bread and cereals.

So what's missing from the list you just read? Carbohydrates. Technically speaking, there's no such thing as a "carbohydrate deficiency." Humans can survive without them. We'll die without essential nutrients that can only be obtained from protein and fat, but life without carbs would merely be inconvenient and (probably) unpleasant. You can get the most important nutrients carbohydrate-rich foods offer—fiber, vitamin C, and calcium—from supplements.

But unless you have a medical reason, it makes little sense to avoid carbs entirely. A diet that's more or less balanced in the three major macronutrients—protein, fat, carbs—is a good choice for almost everyone who works out with the goal of getting leaner.

For the rest of this chapter, let's look at each macronutrient in more detail.

Protein

Bodybuilders, athletes, muscleheads, and gym rats tend to be maximalists when it comes to dietary protein. The academically minded like to argue over how much your body can actually use to build muscle. And militant anti-meat types like to point to the minimum needed to prevent deficiency.

For entertainment value, if nothing else, let's start with that minimum.

According to the official Dietary Reference Intakes, calculated by the U.S. Institute of Medicine, an adult weighing 154 pounds would need just 56 grams of protein a day. That's 0.8 grams per kilogram of body weight, if you want to run your own numbers. (A kilogram is 2.2 pounds.) For a 125-pound woman, it's 45 grams. For a 180-pounder like me, the DRI is 65 grams. Cutting my daily intake down to that level would be a hell of a trick, considering that my usual breakfast has 42 grams all by itself. Your body can survive at this level because it seems to be able to recycle its own protein, in the absence of new protein from your meals.

Fun to know? Sure. Useful? Let me put it this way: A lot of people start a new program with a "before" picture. If you were to take a picture of yourself today, and then eat this minuscule amount of protein for the next three months while doing Alwyn's workouts, your "before" picture would look dramatically better than the picture you take ninety days from now. You'd lose muscle, and possibly gain fat as well. Your body wouldn't be able to replace the muscle protein broken down by your workouts, and your metabolism would probably slow down as well.

And, to be honest, it's all kind of academic anyway; if you eat enough calories to get through Alwyn's workouts, it would be nearly impossible to take in protein at the DRI minimum. You'd have to survive on a diet of fruit, vegetables, and Wonder Bread. Just about everything else in our food chain has some protein in it.

Now to the research. The consensus today is that athletes need about twice the DRI, or 1.6 grams of protein per kilogram of body weight per day. For a 154-pound adult, that would be 112 grams. For me, it would be 131. For a 125-pound woman, it would be 91.

You can hit these levels by accident with a clean and balanced diet. Consider this bare-bones daily menu:

Meal	Contents	Protein grams	Calories
Breakfast	2 eggs 1 slice whole-wheat toast Coffee with half-and-half	17	260
Snack	1 cup cottage cheese	30	200
Lunch	Subway 6-inch turkey breast sandwich	18	280
Snack	Handful of cashews (¼ cup)	5	165
Dinner	Roasted chicken breast Small dinner salad	40	300

We can all agree that this is a tiny amount of food—about 1,200 calories, depending on how you calculate the serving sizes. (These numbers come from a variety of sources, including the USDA database; with some I rounded up and down a little.) But even this starvation diet gives you 110 grams of protein.

Now let's look at a meal plan for a musclehead:

Meal	Contents	Protein grams	Calories
Breakfast	Perkins Build-Your-Own Omelet with 3 eggs, vegetables, and cheese 2 slices whole-wheat toast Coffee with half and half	50	970
Snack	2 tablespoons peanut butter 1 apple	8	300
Lunch	Subway 12-inch turkey breast sandwich	35	450
Snack	Post-workout protein shake 1 banana	40	420
Dinner	8-ounce sirloin steak Broccoli Baked potato	56	670

Some caveats apply. You never know what you're getting in a restaurant, and with a steak, it's really difficult to assess exactly how much meat you have left once you trim the fat and cook it to your taste.

With that said, my ballpark figures tell us we're now looking at about 2,800 calories, with 189 grams of protein (about 27 percent of total calories). I would gain weight if I consistently ate this much food in a day, but for some of the bigger guys reading this, it might be a viable fat-loss diet. Either way, my point stands: It's easy to get all the protein your body would ever need with a fairly simple, convenient, and relatively clean diet.

Should you get more protein than you need? I think there are three good arguments for doing exactly that:

1. Protein increases satiety

The more protein you eat, the less hungry you are for everything else. Swap out some of the carbs and fat in your diet for the same amount of energy in the form of protein, and you'll feel fuller for a longer time after that meal. This effect may even out over time, as your body gets used to it, but in the short term you'll almost certainly benefit from having more protein, fewer carbs, and less fat.

2. Protein increases metabolism

Eating is inefficient. A certain percentage of the calories in each meal are burned off during digestion. This is called the thermic effect of food, or TEF. The TEF for protein is close to 25 percent, far higher than for carbs (6 to 8 percent) or fat (2 to 3 percent).

About 10 percent of your metabolism—the calories you burn each day—comes from TEF. If you eat more protein and less of something else, your metabolism should speed up by a few calories a day.

3. Protein increases muscle mass

Yes, the simple act of eating more protein increases the amount of protein in your muscles. Why? Because that's pretty much the only place your body can store it. It's difficult to turn protein into glucose to use for energy, or into fat for storage. So it leads to higher protein turnover in your muscles—more is broken down, and more is added—with a small net gain in total muscle protein.

Your body also breaks down and builds up muscle tissue at an accelerated rate when you work out with weights. In fact, if you don't supply your muscles with fresh

Minimal Protein, Minimal Life Span?

In a University of Arkansas study published in 2001, a group of men, ages fifty-five to seventy-seven, ate the recommended minimum amount of protein for fourteen weeks—0.8 grams of protein per kilogram of body weight per day. By the end their thigh circumferences had decreased an average of 1.7 centimeters, or about two-thirds of an inch.

No big deal, right? Well, consider this: In a study published in 2009, Danish researchers found that elderly men and women with the thinnest thighs had the highest risk of heart disease and premature death. The magic number for thigh girth—measured right below the gluteal fold—is 55 centimeters, or 21.6 inches. Anything smaller signals higher-than-average risk. The protective benefits of thigh circumference peak at about 60 centimeters (23.5 inches).

The researchers didn't calculate the ratio of fat to muscle in their subjects' legs, but I'll take a wild guess at the implications:

Thigh-muscle mass is a decent stand-in for total-body strength, physical activity, good nutrition, and overall vitality in men, who tend to have little fat in their thighs. For women, girth represents a combination of muscle and fat. Muscle would be a life extender for the same reasons it works for men. But the fat is also important. We know that lower-body fat is cardioprotective, even if a lot of women reading this are engaged in a lifelong battle against it.

Techniques for increasing lower-body fat are beyond my mission here, but in just three words I can tell you how to build bigger and stronger thigh muscles: Do. Alwyn's. Workouts. And don't skimp on the protein.

protein after you lift, you'll end up with a net loss of muscle protein in the hours immediately following your workout. When you do take in that protein, there's a multiplier effect: You add more to your muscles than you would by either lifting without eating or eating without lifting.

Where It Is: Protein

It's a lot easier to find abundant, high-quality protein in animal foods than in plants. That's because meat, eggs, dairy, and fish contain all twenty amino acids, the building blocks of protein. Of these, nine are considered "essential," meaning you need to get them from your food because your body can't make them.

Soy is the only plant-derived protein that has all nine essential amino acids. Nuts, seeds, beans, and whole grains are considered incomplete proteins. (The fact they have any protein at all is a bonus, considering that these foods are loaded with healthy nutrients.) For practical purposes, it doesn't really matter if individual foods offer all or part of the mix of amino acids you need to build muscle. Your body is smart enough to put them together on its own.

Here's a quick rundown of the major categories of protein-rich foods, and how much protein you can expect to find in them.

Food	Amount of protein
Beans	12–17 grams per cup
Beef and pork (lean cuts)	6–7 grams per ounce
Chicken and turkey (boneless and skinless)	6–7 grams per ounce
Cheese	4–10 grams per ounce
Cottage cheese	30 grams per cup
Eggs	6 grams per egg
Fish	6–7 grams per ounce
Green peas (frozen, then cooked)	8 grams per cup
Milk	8 grams per cup (9 per cup for nonfat)
Nuts	5–8 grams per ¼ cup
Peanut butter	4 grams per tablespoon (typical serving size is 2 tablespoons)
Rice, brown or white (cooked)	4–5 grams per cup
Tofu	20 grams per cup
Whole-grain bread or pasta	3–8 grams per serving (although some products go higher than this)

Carbohydrates and Fat

Our perception of these two macronutrients has gone through three major stages since I started writing about fitness and nutrition in 1992:

STAGE 1: CARBS ARE GOOD, FAT IS BAD.

Everyone seemed to believe this. For a journalist like me to write anything else would've been considered blasphemy. The conventional wisdom grew out of three flawed beliefs:

1. Dietary fat causes heart disease.

In any large survey of any industrialized population, it's practically guaranteed that the least healthy people will eat the sloppiest diets, will have the most heart attacks, and will be most likely to die prematurely. But does that mean dietary fat itself is a killer, or that a careless diet filled with cheap, greasy food is merely correlated with a bunch of things known to have negative consequences?

The Nurses' Health Study, a survey of more than 75,000 women that began in 1976, looked at the connection between fat and heart disease. When the researchers factored out all the things that we know are associated with poor health—age, smoking, family history of heart disease, lack of physical activity, and body size, to name just a few—they found something that's kind of amazing: The women who ate the most fat (44 percent of the total calories in their diet) had slightly *lower* rates of heart disease than the women who ate the least (28 percent of total calories).

The same was true with saturated fat, which was once universally described as "artery clogging."

There were only two statistically significant links between fat and heart disease: Trans fats, the man-made fats that are often added to baked goods and other highly processed foods, were linked to a higher risk. And polyunsaturated fats, found in just about everything from eggs to corn oil, were linked to a lower risk. Neither of these correlations was considered a surprise when the study came out in 2005.

The big take-away message? Don't eat fried Twinkies, and stop looking for simple solutions to a problem as complex as heart disease.

2. Fat makes you fat.

This one is actually true, although it's only part of the story. I noted earlier that fat has a very low thermic effect; just 2 to 3 percent of fat calories burn off during digestion. All the rest is used for energy, or stored for future use. And you know where those storage bins are located. Bellies. Thighs. Buttocks. Your body has a limitless capacity to store fat. It's like sculpting your body in reverse. Fat will turn men's pecs into man-boobs and women's triceps into water wings, and will transform anyone's chin from singular to plural.

But it will only do this if you're eating too much. Maintain energy balance, in which the calories coming in match the calories going out, and you don't have to worry about the percentage of calories from fat. Your body will use the carbs and fat you eat for energy. Eat less than you need for energy balance, and your body will use stored fat to make up the difference. This is the part of the process where those love handles, saddlebags, and redundant chins go back where they came from.

When you overeat, on the other hand, your body will store the excess calories. It'll preferentially use the carbs in your diet for energy, since that's the easiest thing to do. And it'll send the fat it doesn't need into storage because, again, it's the easiest thing to do. It can turn carbs or even protein to fat, but it's not quite so easy, so it doesn't happen as often.

The solution here is simple enough: Don't overeat, and you don't have to worry about your body storing fat.

3. Fat has very little functional or nutritional value.

This one is simply ridiculous, and I don't think anyone believes it anymore. About 60 percent of the calories our bodies burn at rest come from fat. The only time fat isn't our preferred source of energy is when we're exercising; the harder you work out, the higher the percentage of glucose your body uses. All-out exercise burns almost 100 percent carbohydrates, but that's a meaningless variable in terms of your overall energy balance. You only exercise at that level for a few seconds at a time, and as soon as you finish you go back to burning a higher percentage of fat calories.

So that's the functional value of dietary fat. (For now, I'll leave aside the role it plays in satiety.) The nutritional value is equally clear: As I noted earlier, vitamins A, D, E, and K are fat-soluble, meaning we need some fat in our diet to put them to use. I'll say more about fat later in this chapter; for now, let's just say that a healthy diet includes fat, and there's very little dispute about this point.

STAGE 2: CARBS ARE BAD, FAT IS GOOD.

Books like *The Zone, Dr. Atkins' New Diet Revolution, Protein Power,* and *The South Beach Diet* changed our view of carbohydrates. (I like to think that my first book, *The Testosterone Advantage Plan,* played a small role in the paradigm shift, but I'd be hard-pressed to back that up with empirical data.) It was in many ways the mirror image of the original argument against fat. The guilt-by-timeline argument went something like this:

1. The U.S. government in the 1970s advocated a low-fat diet, at the same time it was offering new incentives to farmers who planted corn. These policy decisions led to a food chain suddenly overflowing with cheap and increasingly palatable low-fat foods, which Americans proceeded to overeat at unprecedented levels.
2. As Americans got fatter, the government and official nutrition-advocacy groups doubled down on the low-fat message, encouraging us to cut back on fat wherever we could. These messages sent us out in search of even more low-fat food, which made us even fatter.
3. Since the rise in obesity coincided with the message to eat carbs instead of fat, a lot of people concluded that low-fat diets must have made us fat.

The theoretical mechanism for this fat-building machine is insulin. You already know that insulin is a powerful storage hormone. It also has a role in regulating appetite. When everything is working properly, the rise in blood sugar following a meal is accompanied by a rise in insulin, which finds places to store the food—in your muscles, if protein and glucose are needed there; in your liver, where some fat and glucose are kept in reserve; and in your fat cells, if there's a surplus of energy. Insulin's appetite-suppressing signals to your brain should prevent you from feeling hungry while this is going on.

However, we know that obesity is often accompanied by insulin resistance, a condition in which your body stops responding to the hormone's signals. The result is too much blood sugar floating around with no place to go, high blood pressure, and a higher risk for heart disease. But is insulin resistance a *cause* of obesity, or something that develops because you're obese? Put another way: Does insulin, which responds most powerfully to meals high in carbs, make people fat? Or do the excess calories in those high-carb meals make people fat, with insulin acting more like a neutral arbiter?

If the answer to the first question is yes, then all the people touting low-carb diets are correct, and all the people who advocated low-fat diets, which are necessarily high in carbs, are guilty of plus-sizing an entire generation of Americans.

Pretty high stakes, wouldn't you say?

Indeed, people on low-carb diets do seem to lose weight faster and more reliably than people on other types of diets. But the gap between low-carb and low-fat diets isn't really all that dramatic, and the studies don't uniformly present insulin as the bad guy.

One of my favorites was conducted by Christopher Gardner and colleagues at Stanford University. Called the A to Z Weight Loss Study, it assessed the effects of four archetypal diets on overweight women:

- Atkins (extreme low-carb)
- Zone (moderate low-carb)
- LEARN (moderate low-fat)
- Ornish (extreme low-fat)

The results of the study are interesting enough: Women on the Atkins diet lost an average of 10 pounds in 12 months, as opposed to 6 pounds on LEARN, 5 pounds on Ornish, and 4 pounds for those who dared to enter the Zone. Other studies have shown closer results, and those are interesting as well. But the main reason I like this one so much is because of the author's cheerfully acknowledged bias. In an hour-plus video lecture that's available on YouTube, he says that he's a twenty-five-year vegetarian who started out with absolutely no interest in comparing popular diets. He was pushed in that direction because no matter how hard he tried to interest students in his preferred research topics, including soy and garlic, the first questions he heard inevitably concerned low-carb, meat-heavy diets.

So Gardner let the Wookiee win, and put together a serious, well-designed, and carefully executed twelve-month study. It was published in 2007 in the *Journal of the American Medical Association.*

The study shows how difficult it is for anyone to stick to an extreme diet. Ornish says just 10 percent of daily calories should come from fat, while Atkins recommends just 50 grams of "net" carbs a day (total carbs minus fiber) during the major weight-loss phase. Those 50 grams would provide 200 calories, or about 13 percent of a 1,500-calorie diet. By the end of the study, the Atkins dieters were getting about a third of their calories from carbs, while the Ornish eaters were getting 29 percent fat. When people who're sincerely trying to comply overshoot their targets by close to 200 percent, you know the standards are profoundly unrealistic.

One more finding in the study, which gets back to my original point in this section, is that *there were no significant differences* in insulin and blood-sugar levels. All of the diet groups saw modest declines in the amount of insulin circulating in their blood when it was tested first thing in the morning, before they'd eaten breakfast. Three of the four groups saw declines in glucose.

So I think it's important to put insulin back where it belongs in the conversation about weight control and body composition. It's important, but it's not the reason you get fat, and just about any serious attempt to reduce weight will make it work better for you.

STAGE 3: CARBS ARE FOOD, FAT IS FOOD.

This is where I think we are today. Eat too much of anything, and you will gain weight. It doesn't matter if the excess calories come from carbs or fat. When there's an excess, as I noted, your body will choose to use carbs for fuel while storing fat. That doesn't mean carbs make you thin or fat makes you fat, as most of us believed a couple decades ago, or that carbs make you fat and fat keeps you thin, as many now believe.

Food is nourishment, food is fuel, food is a drugstore, and food sometimes is fun or even seductive. Food can make you leaner or fatter, give you energy or take it away, improve your health or rob you of it, make you distinctively sexy or forgettably plain. In most cases, the exact same foods can bestow all those benefits or present all those risks. It's not the food that's good or bad. It's how you use it.

Where They Are: Carbohydrates

Carbs are found almost entirely in plant foods. (Milk is the only animal food that contains carbohydrates.) It's easiest to think of carbs in terms of two major categories: sugars and starches. Here are the sugars:

Fructose, found in fruit and vegetables, is the sweetest-tasting sugar by a wide margin.

Sucrose is a combination of glucose and fructose that's found in sugarcane, beets, peaches, and pineapple. It's also found on tables, in little packets, which is why it's usually referred to as "table sugar."

Lactose, a combination of glucose and another sugar called galactose, is found in milk, and has less than one-tenth of the sweetness of fructose.

Maltose is found in germinating grains. As you can guess by the name, it's a key component of beer brewing, which means it holds a special place in the hearts of most of the men reading this.

Fiber also falls into the sugar category, although its calories are negligible because your body can't use them for energy.

Starches are more complex molecules that usually coexist with sugars in plant foods. It's hard for your body to use many sources of starch without cooking or otherwise processing them. That's why grains and tubers, a category of root vegetables that includes potatoes and yams, are relatively late arrivals to our food chain. For most of human evolution, animals ate grasses and roots and other sources of starch, while our ancestors ate fruit, nuts, and any animals they could kill or steal from other predators.

Nobody's quite sure when humans started cooking food. Some argue it was nearly 2 million years ago, although the more conventional view suggests humans started using hearths a mere 250,000 years before the Food Channel launched. If it was the latter date, it explains why our brains started getting bigger while our teeth got smaller about that time. We had more nutrients available, thanks to our ability to cook meat and easy-to-find but hard-to-digest wild tubers, and we didn't need to work so hard to chew the food. (I don't know what a raw root vegetable tasted like in ancient Africa, but I can't imagine it was something our Paleolithic human ancestors looked forward to eating.)

Cooking changed early humans in profound ways. They formed family and communal groups. Females got bigger while males stayed about the same size. Babies got bigger and fatter, and spent more time helplessly dependent on their mothers for food and protection. (This might explain why women grew larger, relative to the men of their era.) Those extra calories and nutrients now accessible in cooked food literally made us what we are today.

Tubers weren't the only fresh source of starches available to evolving humans. New archaeological findings suggest that cereal grains were gathered and processed 100,000 years ago.

The next big leap in food consumption came during the Neolithic period, roughly ten thousand years ago (give or take a few millennia). That's when humans developed agriculture. Wheat is thought to be the first cultivated crop in the Middle East, followed by barley, peas, and beans. In the Far East, it was rice, followed eventually by soybeans. In Africa, rice and sorghum. And in the Americas, it was maize—what we now call corn—that started things off, followed by potatoes, tomatoes, and peppers.

What seemed like a solution to the problem of nutritional uncertainty—the ability to grow and harvest far more starchy carbs than we could eat—created its own set of problems. It's also when the words "nasty, brutish, and short" could reasonably describe human existence. People lived in ever-bigger communities, and society eventually stratified into haves and have-nots. Infectious diseases arose. Dependence on a single crop meant that failure of that crop could have disastrous consequences. Life expectancy dropped, and physical stature—which should have risen with the systematic production of calorie-rich food—consistently fell as cities got bigger and social inequality more pronounced. In hard times the best food stayed with the wealthiest people, and everyone else got deficiencies and diseases.

But when people had more room to grow, and more freedom to produce or acquire food, they got taller. At the time of the Revolutionary War, Americans were on average three inches taller than Europeans. The average white male in the early United States was five feet, nine inches tall—just a half-inch shorter than his counterpart today. The benefits of North American life extended to everyone, including the slaves who never wanted to be here, and Indian tribes who never requested the pleasure of my forebears' company. Men of the northern Cheyenne tribe were the tallest in the world in the late nineteenth century. They were nearly five-feet-ten on average, or about as tall as we are now.

So what does this have to do with starch? Take the Cheyenne: Most of their diet was bison and berries. Protein, fat, and sugar, with the sugar accompanied by antioxidants and other health-promoting micronutrients. The tradeoff for today's abundant and cheap sources of highly refined starches—mostly wheat, rice, and corn—is that we're getting wider instead of taller. Just as we've conquered diseases of pestilence, we've created diseases of abundance. You know the roll call: obesity, heart disease, cancer, diabetes.

The hell of it is, there's nothing wrong with starches as part of the human diet. Whole grains, like fruits and vegetables, are associated with a long list of health benefits. The problem is with the volume of the food, and how rapidly it breaks down into glucose and reaches your bloodstream.

The way that glucose hits your bloodstream, as a gentle trickle or a biblical deluge, matters tremendously. Nutrition researchers call this *glycemic load*, and according to a 2007 editorial in the *Journal of the American College of Cardiology*, it may be the biggest culprit in obesity, diabetes, and heart disease. Glycemic load (GL) is different from *glycemic index*—a term you're probably more familiar with—because it uses the likely serving size of a particular food as its point of reference. Glycemic index (GI) uses 50 grams of everything as its standard.

For example, 50 grams of raw carrots has a GI of 49; it falls into the low-to-moderate range compared to pure glucose, which has a GI of 100. But a medium-size carrot, which weighs 11 grams, has a barely registering GL of 2. Compare that with a blueberry muffin. It has a moderate GI of 59, not a whole lot higher than raw carrots, while its GL is a whopping 28.

Those aren't the only two ways to measure the immediate impact of foods. There's also the *insulin index*, which measures how much insulin is released by any particular food, and the *satiety index*, which measures the extent to which that food leaves you feeling full and satisfied between meals. As you can see from the following chart, it's hard to predict how different foods will rank on all four measures.

A high GI is anything over 70. A high GL is over 20. The insulin index (II) is designed to be comparable to the GI. The satiety index (SI) has its own scale; anything below 100 could be considered a relatively unsatisfying food. Non-dairy animal foods don't have a GI or GL, since they don't have carbs. But they clearly have an impact on insulin and satiety, as you see in the chart.

Food	GI	GL	II	SI
Apple	38	6	59	197
Baked beans	40	6	120	168
Banana	52	12	81	118
Beef	n/a	n/a	51	176
Bread, white	73	10	100	100
Bread, whole-grain	71	9	96	157
Doughnuts	76	15	74	68
Eggs	n/a	n/a	31	150
Ice cream	57	6	89	96
Pasta, brown	37	27	40	188
Pasta, white	44	18	40	119
Potato (baked)	85	26	121	323
Rice, brown	55	16	62	132
Rice, white	87	36	79	138

White bread is predictably high on the glycemic and insulin measures, and low in terms of satiety. You can see that whole-grain bread is just slightly better across the board. Ice cream and baked beans have low glycemic loads, but trigger extremely high insulin reactions. Then they diverge from each other on satiety: Beans have a decent rating, but ice cream is only slightly more appetite-suppressing than a doughnut.

For extremes, it's hard to beat the baked potato. Despite a sky-high glycemic load and insulin index, it has the highest satiety index measured. So in exchange for rapid digestion, there's a long interval before you get hungry again.

Nutritionists are quick to point out that these indices don't really reflect how people actually eat food. You probably wouldn't eat a baked potato by itself. If you combine it with a nice steak, the beef would moderate the insulin response to the potato. And since both foods rank high on the satiety index, you have to think you'll still feel full for a long time between meals.

Before I move on to fat, let's look at one more carb-related topic: fiber.

You know it's good for you, so I won't list every known benefit. Two big ones: It helps you feel full longer between meals, and provides a conditioning stimulus to your digestive system—a workout for the smooth muscles of your intestines and colon.

It also, as you know, makes you regular, a benefit we take for granted now. But just a century ago, constipation was a major public-health issue. As James C. Whorton wrote in a book called *Inner Hygiene*, "Civilization encourages constipation." Machine processing of wheat began in the late nineteenth century in Europe, and for the first time it was possible to remove all the unstable compounds from flour and create a long-lasting, cheap, and highly portable calorie-delivery system. Fiber-free white flour became a staple in our diets, and our bowels paid the price. Health gurus in the late nineteenth and early twentieth centuries railed against processed foods. One of them, Bernarr Macfadden, even campaigned for president on a platform that highlighted his antipathy to white bread. Macfadden and others touted the benefits of colon cleansing, called "the water cure."

The two main categories of fiber are soluble and insoluble. Soluble fiber includes the pectin in apples and oats, which bulks up solid waste in your intestines and slows down its transit to the municipal sewer system. Insoluble fiber, such as the bran from whole grains, speeds things up.

Here's a quick look at some fiber-rich foods. Your target is 20 to 35 grams a day—the low end is for petite women and the high end is for large guys. No matter your size or gender, you'd have to eat a lot of fiber before the excess becomes a problem.

Food	Serving size	Fiber grams	Calories
Apple	1	3.7	138
Avocado	1	10	324
Banana	1	2.8	105
Black beans, cooked	1 cup	15	227
Bread, whole wheat	1 slice	2	70
Broccoli or cauliflower	1 cup	2.5	24
Oatmeal, cooked	1 cup	4	150
Orange	1	3.1	62
Peas, split, cooked	1 cup	16	230
Prunes	10	6	201
Raisins	1 cup (packed)	6.6	488
Raspberries	1 cup	8.4	61
Rice, brown, cooked	1 cup	3.5	350

You're probably surprised to see that most fruits and vegetables don't have all that much fiber until you get into multiple servings. In a clean diet, you can't go wrong with legumes like beans and peas—lots of fiber, and lots of protein, with relatively few total calories.

But you can do even better than that, if you're willing to start the day with some processed food. I have two cups of Kashi Go Lean cereal for breakfast each day, which give me 20 grams of fiber. And that's nothing compared to Fiber One cereal. One cup gives you 28 grams, with just 120 calories.

Where It Is: Fat

When we talk about dietary fats, we have an unfortunate tendency to assign to them magical qualities, positive and negative, that far exceed their biological distinctions. You've probably seen books and articles in which fats are arranged in these five categories:

- saturated
- monounsaturated
- omega-6 polyunsaturated
- omega-3 polyunsaturated
- trans

All of these are a type of fat called triglycerides. The "glyceride" part comes from glycerol, which is actually a type of carbohydrate—sugar alcohol, to be precise. That would be a really entertaining factoid if triglycerides had any intoxicating qualities, which, alas, they don't. The "tri" part comes from three chains of carbon atoms. The other components are hydrogen atoms, which attach to the carbons. A fat is "saturated" if it has all the hydrogen atoms it can hold. It's "monounsaturated" if it's missing one hydrogen, and "polyunsaturated" if it's missing two or more.

If you add hydrogen atoms to an unsaturated fat—a process called "hydrogenation," appropriately enough—you get a "trans" fat, meaning it's a fat made from spare parts.

Your body can also play that game, making saturated or monounsaturated fats from scratch, since there's no shortage of the components floating around inside you. The two it can't make are both polyunsaturated: linoleic acid, an omega-6 fat, and linolenic acid, an omega-3.

I'm going to assume that most of you, like me, weren't trained in biochemistry or nutrition science. Me, I barely passed Chemistry I in high school. So when I look at carbon and hydrogen combinations that barely differ from each other in structure, or try to remember whether "linoleic" or "linolenic" is the one found in mayonnaise (answer: linoleic), I ask what I think is a logical question: Do we really need to make such a *big freakin' deal* out of such small differences?

The answer begins with a slight digression:

Earlier in this chapter, I noted that only trans fats are associated with heart disease as a causative agent. It's instructive to note how those trans fats became part of our food chain.

Some trans fats occur in nature—conjugated linoleic acid (CLA) is one, found in the meat and milk of cud-chewing animals like cattle, sheep, and goats. Kangaroo meat is thought to have the highest concentrations. Different types of CLA have been assigned positive and negative health consequences. On the plus side, they may help reduce body fat and perhaps even prevent cancer. On the downside, there's illness, death, and unnatural cravings for kangaroo meat. Whether CLA is ultimately considered good, bad, or neutral, it's unlikely we'll ever eat enough of it to make a difference. (Unless a cow is raised on a pasture where it can eat grass, its meat and milk will have very little CLA.)

We can't say that about the trans fats created in labs and inserted into our food supply. Americans got their first dose in the early twentieth century, when Procter & Gamble introduced Crisco, a shortening made from cottonseed oil, and popularized it by giving away free cookbooks. Its popularity was understandable; because it was an unsaturated vegetable fat that had been chemically altered to make it behave like a saturated animal fat, it could replace butter or lard in baking. Shortening was cheaper and more stable than those animal fats, and gave baked goods a longer shelf life.

I don't think anyone in the first half of the 1900s saw Crisco as a healthy alternative. However, in the second half of the century, another trans-fat product called "oleomargarine" was sold as exactly that. (When I was growing up in the 1960s, some adults still called it "oleo," although most people by then just called it "margarine.") Doctors and nutrition professionals were convinced that saturated fat caused heart disease, and the public followed their lead. The nadir came in the 1980s, when an organization called Center for Science in the Public Interest (CSPI) pressured fast-food restaurants to fill their frying vats with hydrogenated fats instead of the beef fat they used at the time. (Give CSPI credit for being an equal-opportunity scold: When information emerged about the dangers of trans fats, CSPI called a press conference in October 1993 to attack the restaurant chains for taking their advice.)

To review, the food industry created an entire category of fake fats to replace a real fat that we now know wasn't much of a threat to begin with. So we can conclude, simply enough, that fake fats are bad.

But what about those structural differences among the real fats? Are they *really* that different?

Short answer: Sure, they're different. (As for what we need to worry about, that's a pretty short list, which I'll explain in a moment.) We know, for example, that calories from some fats tend to get used faster than others. A study published in 2000 in the *American Journal of Clinical Nutrition* found that about 40 percent of a saturated fat called lauric acid was metabolized in the nine hours following consumption. That compares with 27 percent of linolenic acid (an omega-3 fat found in flaxseeds and flaxseed oil), 20 percent for linoleic acid (an omega-6 fat found in soybean oil), 18 percent for oleic acid (a monounsaturated fat found in olive oil), and just 13 percent for stearic acid (a saturated fat found in beef and chocolate).

So lauric acid sounds like a pretty good choice. And I'm sure it is. But good luck finding a lot of it in anything other than pure coconut oil.

As for the other fats I mentioned, they're everywhere. Take butter, for example. A tablespoon has 11.5 grams of fat, including more than 7 grams that are saturated. Bad, right? Not really. Just 12 percent of the fat in butter comes from slow-to-metabolize stearic acid. The rest of the saturated fat, including a teeny bit of lauric acid, has shorter chains of carbon atoms, meaning they metabolize faster. It also has 3 grams of monounsaturated fat and about a gram of polyunsaturated fat for good measure.

Now we're getting back to all that headache-inducing chemistry, but it's in the service of an important point: When we eat foods that are reasonably close to their natural state—and butter is just a couple steps removed from cow's milk, straight from the teat—we're eating a mix of fats. I could hit you with zillions of studies showing what each fat does or doesn't do, but I don't think it's worth the trouble to me, or the confusion for you. Most of the fat-rich foods nature provides for us include all the major types, plus lots of variation within those types. Butter has thirteen different fats. Ground beef has ten. An egg has at least trace amounts of fifteen. Milk has eleven.

If you eat a mix of animal and plant foods, you naturally get a mix of fats, and you don't have to worry about which particular ones are the most bioactive. It's only when you eat a lot of processed junk—chips, fast food, baked desserts—that you risk an overload of one particular type of fat relative to the others.

The worst-case scenario is an imbalance of the two essential fats—omega-6 and omega-3. Soybean oil, rich in omega-6 linoleic acid, is now the most ubiquitous fat in the modern food chain. And there's hardly any omega-3 left in our food, unless you eat a lot of fish, walnuts, and grass-fed beef.

A study published in *Psychosomatic Medicine* highlighted the dangers of an imbalanced ratio of omega-6 to omega-3 fats. Pre-agriculture, the ratio in human diets was thought to be 2 to 1 or 3 to 1. That is, two or three times as much omega-6. But today, the ratio is more like 15 to 1. In the study, the researchers found that the higher the ratio in their subjects (average age: sixty-seven), the greater their risk of depression, and the more markers of inflammation they had circulating through their blood. Those with major depression had an average ratio of 18 to 1. (This was after they dropped a subject whose blood showed a 168 to 1 mix and another outlier with a relatively healthy 49 to 1.) The ratio for those without depression was 13.5 to 1.

We also know that omega-6 fats are linked to higher levels of inflammation, and that inflammation is linked to heart disease and who knows how many other problems.

That's why the best advice right now is to actively seek out omega-3 fat, either through fatty fish like salmon, or through supplements like fish-oil pills. At the same time, we need to avoid excessive omega-6 fats, especially processed foods that contain soybean, cottonseed, corn, or safflower oils.

The following chart shows some common foods and their mix of the major categories of fats.

Food	Serving size	Calories	Total fat (grams)	Sat (grams)	MUFA (grams)	n-6 (grams)	n-3 (grams)
Avocado	1	218	20	3	13	2	trace
Butter	1 tbsp	102	11.5	7.5	3	0.5	trace
Chicken, dark meat	6 oz*	274	12	3.5	4.5	2.5	0.5
Egg	1	72	5	1.5	2	1	trace
Ground beef	4 oz	281	17	7	7.5	0.5	trace
Milk (whole)	1 cup	146	8	5.5	2	trace	trace
Olive oil	1 tbsp	119	13.5	2	10	1.5	trace
Peanut butter	2 tbsp	188	16	3.5	8	4.5	trace
Salmon	6 oz	236	7	2	3	trace	2
Walnuts	¼ cup	196	20	2	3	11	3

Key: Sat = saturated; MUFA = monounsaturated; n-6 = omega-6 polyunsaturated; n-3 = omega-3 polyunsaturated
*Boneless and skinless.

The numbers in the four right-hand columns won't always add up to equal the total fat grams, due to rounding and other nuances. Because these numbers came from several sources, all of which disagree with each other in minor ways, they may not reflect exactly what you had for dinner last night. But, as I've argued in this section, a gram of this or that totally doesn't matter. It's what you have habitually for months and years that makes a difference.

"We Who Are About to Diet Salute You!"

I'VE MET A LOT of truly smart, passionate people in my time as a fitness journalist, along with some genuine dummies. Some of the smartest and many of the dimmest people share a curious distinction: They're the most certain about the superiority of the extreme diet and workout programs they advocate. The harder the programs are to implement and adhere to, the more *impractical* the programs are for most normal people, the more they believe in them.

I used to assume that serious and driven people, whether they're advocates or end users, gravitated toward these programs because of their difficulty. To these men and women, "impractical" and "extreme" are code for "only the strong-willed can pull this off; the rest of you just keep doing whatever it is that made you weak and fat."

But with age, experience, and perspective, I figured out a different reason why the most grueling and restrictive regimens find so many advocates: If they don't work, it's always the *person* who fails, never the *system*. The system is perfect. If the person can't adhere to a diet that's just 10 percent fat or carbohydrates, it's not the diet that's flawed. It's the dieter. If the exerciser can't run far enough, or lift often enough, or do either at a high enough intensity to get the promised results, don't blame the trainer who created the system. The trainee just doesn't have what it takes.

That's why my books promote a relatively simple diet, with a balance of protein, carbs, and fat. And it's why Alwyn creates workouts for people who get to the gym two or three times a week, rather than four or five. More complicated, restrictive, or demanding plans might get better results, but fewer people would benefit from them.

Which brings me to this rule:

NEW RULE #17 • Don't do a complicated intervention until you've tried all the simple ones.

Readers of my books have taught me that no one ever knows exactly which intervention is going to work until they try it. One reader told me he lost more than twenty pounds straight off his gut when he quit drinking beer every night. The advice to not drink beer was just one line in one book, but for him it was the change that made more difference than all the others combined.

Would that tactic work for everyone? Of course not. (And in the case of the stop-drinking-beer advice, several readers told me it was a deal-breaker; even if it was guaranteed to work, they just didn't want to give up their Guinness.) It simply happened to be the right advice for him at a moment when he was ready to act on it. I could've given him advice about following infinitely complex nutrition plans, but they probably wouldn't have worked nearly as well as his decision not to drink beer.

In the fitness world, the experts have a line that goes something like this: "Don't talk to me about supplements if you're still eating Big Macs." I've heard dozens of variations on that admonition from fitness and nutrition professionals. All are making essentially the same point, which is that you need to master the simple stuff before you'll get anything out of the most complex diet and fitness strategies. If you don't exercise at all, you don't need an advanced bodybuilding program. You need to get off your ass and work out. If you eat what you want when you want, with no dietary discipline, you don't need to know which protein supplement is best. You need to stop eating crap.

In this chapter I'll describe five levels of dietary intervention. Most readers will laugh at the ridiculously obvious advice in Level One, and I assume some readers are already maxed out at Level Four. You decide which level fits your experience, ambition, and comfort level.

LEVEL ONE: STOP BEING A MORON

These admonitions are the absolute baseline for someone reading a fitness book, especially one that emphasizes the waistline. If we were talking about baseball, and you were a pitcher, this would be the part of the program where the coach says, "Just throw strikes." You can't expect to make much progress toward a leaner physique without controlling these basic aspects of your diet.

1. Clean up your act.

When things that are typically dipped into other things are a major source of your daily energy intake, you must stop eating both things. No chips. No dip. No cookies or cakes. If you're going to have a treat, make sure it's your favorite thing, and make sure it's finite. A single candy bar. A single slice of cake. Whatever it is, it starts and stops with that indulgence. One and done.

2. Limit fast food.

You don't have to cut out all fast food, but you shouldn't hear "would you like fries with that?" more than once a week.

3. Eliminate almost all calorie-containing beverages.

If you drink non-diet soda, cut back as much as you can, as fast as you can, with the goal of reaching zero Cokes, Sprites, and Mountain Dews. Limit your beer consumption. And stop with the damned sports drinks. Honestly, do you think Gatorade was invented with you and your workouts in mind?

There's one exception: milk. Studies at McMaster University in Ontario found that young women who drank nonfat milk immediately after strength training, and then again one hour later, built more muscle and lost more fat than a control group that lifted but didn't drink milk afterward. (The control group was given an all-carbohydrate drink instead.) The milk drinkers also gained more strength.

With young men, the researchers found that milk led to greater gains in muscle size and greater losses of body fat, although strength wasn't affected. This study used three groups: One drank dairy milk post-workout. Another got soy milk, and the third got the carbohydrate-only drink. Dairy outperformed soy in muscle gains and fat loss.

The researchers speculate that milk works better for fat loss because of the calcium found in dairy products; a substantial body of research supports the idea. So if you're going to drink anything that contains calories, milk is your best choice, assuming you aren't lactose-intolerant. You might want to limit it to pre- and/or post-workout drinks, when your body can make the best use of its protein and carbs.

4. Pay attention to your urges.

Did you have seconds on dessert because you still felt hungry? Or because you always have seconds? Did you have six beers with your buddies because you can't enjoy yourself with only five beers? Or did you just do it out of habit? If you know you're eating or drinking something that's counterproductive to your goals, you should at the very least understand why you're doing it, and ask yourself how much you truly need to keep doing it.

LEVEL TWO: GET ON THE CLOCK

The fancy name for these interventions is "temporal nutrition." Most of us refer to them as "nutrient timing." You probably recognize them as "common sense." You won't find anything obscure or daunting at this level; in fact, it's not unusual to see this advice on the home page of Yahoo! or AOL.

1. Eat breakfast.

I'll be honest: I can't say for certain that eating a substantial breakfast improves your body composition. But I've never met a nutrition professional willing to say it doesn't matter. Those who eat breakfast tend to be leaner than those who don't. The reverse is also true: Those who skip breakfast tend to be heavier.

Just to pick one example, a study of young women in college found that 48 percent of obese women and 40 percent of overweight women had tried skipping breakfast to help them lose weight, while just 27 percent of the normal-weight students had done this. (A woman who's five-foot-four, 145 pounds, would just hit the cutoff for "normal" weight. At 175 and above, she'd be considered "obese." "Overweight" would be anything over 145 but under 175.)

Are overweight and obese people more likely to skip breakfast out of desperation, or is breakfast-skipping part of the pattern of behaviors that led to excess weight in the first place? I don't think anyone can say. But just about everyone agrees that the correlations are pretty strong. Eat a good breakfast, and you're more likely to be lean than the person who skips breakfast.

2. Eat every four hours.

The question of meal frequency isn't controversial in musclehead circles. Eat five or six meals and snacks a day. Why? Works for us. Next question.

It's hard to come up with proof that this works better than three or four meals a day. We know that for men, eating more often is correlated with having less body fat. With women, it's more nuanced. Those who eat more meals also eat more total calories, but they don't weigh more. A 2008 study in the *American Journal of Clinical Nutrition* found that women who eat more often also exercise more and eat more protein and carbs. Because of that, they're leaner.

You can go around in circles all day on this, but in practice, eating five or six meals and snacks a day seems to work better for people like us, who exercise with the goal of being leaner.

The prescription: Eat a good breakfast, and then eat a meal or snack four hours later. As I suggested in Chapter 14, a meal should keep hunger at bay for four hours, while a snack should tide you over for two hours. So if you eat breakfast at six a.m. and lunch at noon, you should plan on having a snack at ten a.m. to bridge the gap between meals.

If you've tried this and it didn't work for you, I suggest carrying a notebook around and marking down the time of each meal, as well as the first noticeable hunger pang after the meal. If you find you get hungry at inconvenient times, you can do one of two things:

- Eat more food at the previous meal, or eat different food that's more satiating. Protein and fiber will help. Fat doesn't affect how full you feel around the time of the meal, but it takes longer to digest, so it helps increase the interval between hunger pangs.
- Keep snacks on hand—cashews, peanut butter, or protein bars in your desk, or yogurt or cheese sticks in the office fridge. Any of those should hold you over for a couple hours between meals.

The worst strategy is to ignore hunger between meals. Hunger never really goes away. It just builds up and hits you later, when you're exhausted from your day and may not have the willpower to choose and prepare the best food for your goals.

3. Get serious about pre- and/or post-workout nutrition.

I touched on this in Level One, in the advice to drink milk. For those of us who lift, timed protein intake is the difference between building muscle and merely getting some exercise.

Researchers might argue over how much protein it takes before or after a workout to get a muscle-building benefit, but I don't think anyone dismisses the importance of pre- and/or post-workout nutrition. At this point I think it's beyond dispute.

What might be up in the air for readers is why I keep using that annoying "and/or" sentence construction. The advice for years was to have protein and carbs immediately after a workout. Pre-workout nutrition was rarely more detailed than "make sure you have something in your stomach when you lift."

That changed in 2001 when the research team at the University of Texas Medical Branch in Galveston, led by Kevin Tipton and Robert Wolfe, published a study showing that pre-workout protein produced a stronger muscle-building effect than the same amount of protein taken after a workout. They used 6 grams of essential amino acids—the ones your body can't make, which are also the ones with the most powerful muscle-building qualities—along with 35 grams of carbohydrates in the form of pure glucose.

When they repeated the experiment using 20 grams of whey protein instead of the 6 grams of essential amino acids, they found that there was no difference between pre- and post-workout results. That study was published in 2007. The whole thing came full circle when they published a 2009 study showing that pre-workout protein and carbs didn't do anything at all.

That's why I use "and/or." After years of using post-workout protein shakes, I switched to pre-workout shakes in 2009 and found I was able to stay leaner despite the shorter workouts I described at the beginning of this book. I have no idea if switching from post- to pre- mattered, but it felt like it did. Still, the research is all over the place, and there's no telling what will work best for you. Some in the bodybuilding world recommend both pre- and post-workout shakes. (Some even suggest drinking some liquid protein during the workout, as well as before and after.)

I don't see the point in having more than one shake, unless you're in serious bulking-up mode. Whether to have it before or after is something you'll need to figure out on your own.

Are Protein Supplements Necessary?

I'm as big a fan of protein powders as you'll find among those with no financial ties to the supplement industry. To me, they aren't really a supplement; I see them as food—processed, yes, but extremely convenient and useful. Still, I can't argue that they're necessary. Real food—especially milk—should give your muscles the amino acids they need to recover from workouts and come back bigger and stronger.

Most protein supplements are made from milk proteins. Some use whey alone, and others use a combination of whey and casein. The advantage of whey is that it digests fast, but a 2006 study in the *American Journal of Clinical Nutrition* suggests that might also be a disadvantage. The researchers found that it metabolized too quickly to provide the body with an adequate supply of protein beyond the four-hour mark. Casein digests at a slower rate, and thus supplies muscle-building amino acids for a longer time after a meal.

Complete milk protein is about 80 percent casein and 20 percent whey, and in this case nature seems to have gotten it right. So if you're going to use a protein supplement—and I certainly do, on a daily basis—you might have the best results with one that contains a blend of both milk proteins.

Or just use plain old milk.

LEVEL THREE: QUANTIFY

If you're ready for this level, all of the following should describe you:

- Most of your diet is based on clean, unprocessed foods—lean meat, fish, and poultry; fruits and vegetables; nuts and seeds; dairy and eggs.
- You hardly ever have fast food.
- You eat four to six meals and snacks a day. You've arrived at this number for a reason—it's what works best for you.
- You pay attention to the functional qualities of the food you eat. You understand that you need to have some protein at every meal and almost every snack, and that you need to include fiber-rich fruits and vegetables. (An apple is a perfectly fine snack, despite its lack of protein. You get some fiber, and apples have a high satiety index with a relatively low glycemic load.)
- When you indulge yourself with a lush dessert or a late-afternoon candy bar, you understand what you're doing and why. Maybe you need the quick and unsustainable rush of energy a candy bar provides, or the mood-elevating benefits of a slice of chocolate cake. Or it's Christmas, and having a cookie or two brings back some

of your favorite memories. You're making a conscious choice to eat something that doesn't move you closer to your goal of a leaner physique, rather than simply eating something because it's there.

- Despite your mastery of dietary diligence at Level Two, it's not enough. Maybe you have a lot of weight to lose. Maybe you thrive on order and quantifiable achievement. Maybe you're in terrific shape by normal human standards, but for personal or professional reasons you want to do better than that. Whatever the reason, the fact is that you're ready to move beyond general guidelines to specific numbers.

Your new interventions:

1. Weigh yourself every day.

Construction professionals have a maxim: "measure twice, cut once." The first measurement you need is your weight, along with girth measurements of your waist, hips, upper arms, thighs, or whatever else matters to you. When you're serious about changing your body composition, I recommend weighing yourself daily and measuring your waist once a week. Always do this at the exact same time in the morning, after using the bathroom and before eating.

Why daily weighing? A substantial body of research shows that men and women who weigh themselves more often have better success with weight loss and weight maintenance. You'll see minor weight fluctuations in both directions that don't really mean anything, but if you look at the overall trend—up, down, or sideways—you'll see if you're on the right track.

Weight, of course, isn't the only variable when you're working to reduce body fat, which is why you also need girth measurements. Sometimes the two move together, but sometimes they don't. An absolute beginner, for example, might lose fat and build muscle at the same time, producing a smaller waist with no change in weight. Someone who's been out of the gym for a while might regain lost muscle while losing fat in the first few weeks or months of a new program. But it's rare for someone who's been exercising consistently to lose a visually discernible amount of fat without also reducing weight. A dedicated and experienced gym rat usually has to focus on one or the other.

Girth measurements, in my experience, are a little more unpredictable than scale weight, which is why I suggest taking them less often. You may have some mild inflammation in your arms or legs the day after a serious workout, or find yourself a little bloated around the midsection if your dinner included some food you weren't used to. A month's worth of weekly measurements should give you a better indication of whether you're on the right track.

2. Track your calories for three days.

To make this work, you need to write down everything you eat for three days, including portion sizes, and then figure out how many calories that is. This means measuring everything you eat to the best of your ability. Then go to an online calorie calculator, like the one at fitday.com, add up your total for each day, and calculate the average.

3. Calculate your daily protein intake and macronutrient ratios.

You should get a breakdown of protein, fat, and carbs along with your total calories. If the calculator you use doesn't have that feature, at the very least add up the protein grams in everything you eat. Multiply by four to get the calories from protein, and then divide that number by your total calories to figure out your percentage of calories from protein.

At minimum, you should be eating 0.8 gram of protein per pound of body weight. Most of us round up to a gram per pound. Let's say you weigh 160, and you're currently eating 2,500 calories a day, with 150 grams of protein. That's 600 calories from protein, or 24 percent of your daily intake.

You can calculate fat and carbohydrate totals and percentages the same way. Fat gives you 9 calories per gram, and a gram of carbohydrate is 4 calories. So if you have 100 grams of fat per day, that's 900 calories, or 36 percent of your daily total. That leaves 1,000 calories, which would be 250 grams of carbs, and 40 percent of your daily energy.

Now you know exactly how much you're eating, and the percentage that comes from the three major macronutrients. Weighing yourself daily tells you if you're gaining, losing, or maintaining. You have the information you need to start tweaking your diet, if it needs to be tweaked.

4. Nip and tuck as needed.

I don't recommend making any big, deliberate changes to your calorie intake until you've done Alwyn's workouts for four weeks, and tracked changes to your weight and girth measurements. If you've never tried Alwyn's programs before, you'll probably be surprised by how much effort they take, and how much recovery you'll need in between workouts. By themselves, the workouts will create an energy deficit, assuming you're currently eating a weight-maintenance diet. You need the first four weeks to discover how big an energy deficit they give you.

That doesn't mean you can't fix your starting diet; you can certainly swap protein for fat and carbs, as long as it's more or less an even trade, in terms of total calories. (Again, this assumes you're already eating a mostly clean diet. If you're not, of course you should clean it up wherever you can, even if it means cutting some calories.)

After four weeks, if your body composition isn't improving as fast as you'd like, this is the hierarchy of tweaks, from easiest to hardest:

a. Substitute something with more fiber for some of your habitual food choices. If you eat cereal for breakfast, for example, switch to one with more fiber (and perhaps fewer calories per serving). For dinner, try some dishes with more beans and less of something else.

b. A couple nights a week, instead of a piece of meat or fish with vegetables, make a soup with similar ingredients. (You can find good recipes on the Internet in seconds, as you surely know.) You'll probably end up eating less, but feel at least as full as usual, thanks to the water in the soup.

c. Remove some carbohydrates, particularly those with the highest glycemic load (bread, potatoes, pasta, rice). Reserve high-glycemic-load carbs for breakfast and the immediate post-workout meal. This is trickier than the other steps, since you're now taking out calories that you won't replace.

d. If you eat a lot of fruit, try cutting back to two or three servings a day. Fruit is obviously good for you in a million ways, but calories from bananas and melons do add up. This isn't a long-term strategy, but it might help in the short term.

LEVEL FOUR: CYCLE

Since you burn more calories on the days you do Alwyn's workouts, it makes sense to eat more on those days, and less on the days you don't lift. In *NROL for Women*, we suggested that everyone should do this from the start. That's good advice, and the only reason I put it in Level Four is because it takes some diligence to pull this off. After working out for more than forty years, I can't tell you with any certainty that I eat more on the days I hit the weight room. I probably do, just because I'm hungrier, but I wouldn't bet my life savings on it.

If you're willing to move away from a more or less static eating pattern to one in which you consciously manipulate your energy intake, you might experience a break-through. Or you might not. All I know for sure is that lots of fitness and nutrition professionals recommend it.

1. Cycle calories.

Manipulate calories so you eat more on the days you burn more, when you have a pumped-up metabolism thanks to one of Alwyn's workouts. Then you eat less on the other days, when you're doing less activity and your metabolism will be a bit slower.

"More" could mean a simple pre- or post-workout protein shake. Or it could mean a shake, plus a couple hundred extra calories at the first meal following the workout. But if you go to that extreme, then you also have to cut something from your menu on non-gym days.

If you try this, I recommend an initial seven-day target that matches your current weekly calorie intake. That way you'll know if calorie cycling, by itself, produces a result, or if you need to cycle your calories in a way that produces a net calorie deficit.

2. Cycle carbohydrates.

Same idea, but now you're manipulating carbs along with calories. I don't think there's any one way to cycle carbs, so take this as an introduction to the concept, rather than a definitive guide. You could start with three separate meal plans:

- High-carb day. Eat more bread, pasta, rice, or potatoes than you ordinarily would, and eat as little fat as you can. Eat the normal amount of protein, or even a little less than usual. If you're doing Alwyn's workouts on Monday, Wednesday, and Friday, you can use Monday and Friday as "high" days.
- Medium-carb day. Eat about half the carbs you did on your "high" day. This might be your normal meal plan, or it could be slightly lower-carb than usual. Protein and fat are slightly higher than they were on the high-carb day. You could do this on Wednesday and Saturday.
- Low-carb day. Eat as few carbs as possible, with more protein and fat to make up for some of the calorie deficit. You could try this on Tuesday, Thursday, and Sunday.

Or you can combine the medium- and low-carb days, and eat medium-to-low on the days you don't work out with weights. Another approach is to skip high-carb days, and instead eat medium carbs on training days and low carbs the other days.

As with calorie cycling, it's best to start with a plan that more or less matches the total energy in your current weekly diet. If manipulating daily macronutrients as well as daily carbs doesn't give you the results you want, you can try cutting calories, along with carbs, on your non-workout days.

LEVEL FIVE: GIVE IT A REST

If you're doing everything you can and still not getting what you need, break your diet. Totally. Just forget about it for a couple days.

You aren't doing this out of despair. You're doing it to see how your body reacts. What happens when you suddenly flood your body with calories for a day or two? If you feel incredible, and your muscles suddenly fill out, and your waistline stays more or less the same, then you've learned something important: Your body thrives on a periodic refeed.

I've heard versions of this story several times from bodybuilders. They train six or seven days a week and starve themselves to get as lean as possible for a contest, only to be disappointed by the way their body looks onstage. They go out that night and eat an entire sausage pizza as a reward for their discipline (or a palliative for their suffering). When they wake up the next morning and look in the mirror, they see the body they'd hoped to have the day before, when it mattered.

For obvious reasons, you can't eat a pizza every night and hope to look like someone who never eats any food that ends with a vowel. But as countless bodybuilders have discovered, it's possible to take dietary discipline too far, and end up with a body that's too depleted to look or perform the way you'd hoped.

A refeed can be anything you want it to be. It might be a single cheat meal every few days, or an unfettered pig-out after an extended period of dieting. The only rule is that you do it on purpose, and you stop doing it when you feel that you've learned all you can.

You may discover that you didn't really need a refeed. You learn this lesson when your weight and waistline both bulk up, but your muscles don't look any better.

Like everything else when it comes to nutrition, you never know how your body will react until you try it and find out.

Waisted!

Here's what we know about the effects of alcohol on your waistline:

- Alcohol has calories—7 per gram. Excess calories from any source should make you fatter over time.
- Alcohol also has a very high thermic effect, higher even than protein. Much of the energy you must be twenty-one or older to consume gets lost via digestion.
- Because your body has no place to store alcohol, those calories go to the front of the line during digestion, during which time your body stores fat that it would otherwise use for energy.
- In terms of volume, people who drink the least and those who drink the most tend to be fattest. But people who drink the least also tend to have the lowest education levels and get the least exercise. (Smokers cluster at the two extremes—teetotalers and alcoholics are more likely to smoke than moderate drinkers.)
- Moderate alcohol consumption—a drink or two a day—is associated with a lower risk of insulin resistance. That could help prevent weight gain. Similarly, non-stupid drinking habits are linked to less heart disease and a more potent immune system.
- Overall, frequent drinkers are leaner than abstainers and occasional drinkers.

So what's the take-away message? If you don't drink, should you start? And if you're trying to expose as much of your six-pack as age and genetics will allow, is alcohol your friend or your enemy?

I don't think there's any benefit to drinking more than you already do. If you currently drink a lot, it's certainly better to spread out your weekly consumption, compared to slamming it all down on Saturday night and spending the next six days wishing you hadn't. (Never mind the unlikelihood of someone switching from one pattern to the other; drinking habits don't develop in isolation from other lifestyle choices.)

The open question is whether your waistline will benefit if you drink less than you currently do. Does alcohol have a net-positive metabolic effect? Or would you be better off without the calories? The only way to find out is to try it and see.

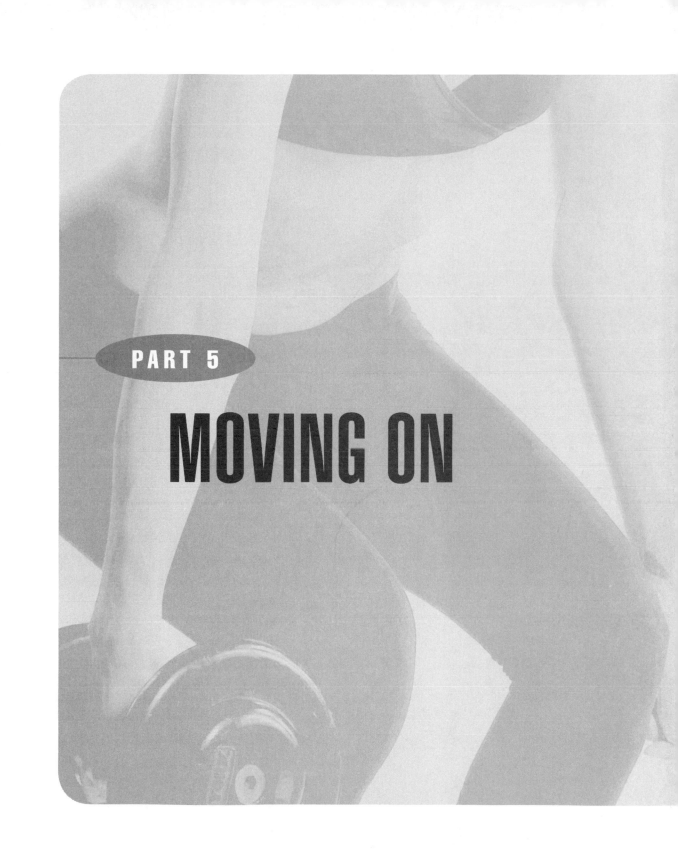

PART 5

MOVING ON

Convergence Training

FOR MOST OF MY LIFE, I've had an open-door policy when it comes to participatory sports. I played every sport I could as a kid, and even as an adult I can't think of many times I've passed up a chance to play anything: golf, beer-league softball, soccer, basketball. I've even tried new sports like lacrosse for no reason beyond the fact that someone brought the equipment and it looked like fun.

The highlight of my rec-sports career, as I mentioned in the Introduction, was the season I played in an over-forty-five baseball league, even though I hadn't been on a team since I was twelve. (Slow-pitch softball doesn't count; compared to baseball, it's the athletic equivalent of hitting a piñata.) Everyone else on my team had at least played through high school. Most had played in college, and a couple had been professionals. All of them had been in adult leagues in recent years.

My season had all the embarrassing moments you'd expect after a forty-year hiatus—dropped fly balls, strikeouts, base-running blunders. But it also had some highlights. I got a couple of clean hits, stole a few bases, scored some runs. Competitively, the results were mixed. But as a fitness pursuit, it was an unqualified success.

Strength coaches like to poke fun at baseball for the sport's somewhat lax conditioning requirements. Unlike soccer or basketball, it's a game that accommodates older, slower, and fatter players at the professional level. But for a middle-aged amateur, a nine-inning game is a workout. When you're in the field, you're constantly moving, or at least preparing to move. When you're on base, if you aren't planning to steal, you at least fake it to distract the pitcher. And when you finally do go for the next base, you cover those ninety feet as fast as you can. A three-hour game ends up involving some of everything: a handful of all-out sprints, a lot of general movement, throwing and catching to warm up before the game and to stay loose between innings, stretching, hitting. Then there's the weather: You might be shivering through a chilly spring rain or melting in the July sun.

No, you won't get six-pack abs from playing baseball, or from any other sport, but you will get tangible benefits. Obviously, you'll burn more calories by playing than you would by watching someone else play on TV. You'll work up a sweat without counting minutes or tracking miles. Less obviously, you'll improve core stability, according to an intriguing study published in 2009 in the *Journal of Strength and Conditioning Research.*

A Danish research group recruited healthy but non-exercising women to either play soccer or run twice a week for sixteen weeks. Their goal was to see if the women playing soccer would develop better protection against "sudden loading" of the upper body—something that might produce a lower-back injury because your lumbar spine is forced out of the neutral position. In an hour of soccer, the researchers calculated an average of 192 sudden-loading challenges for each player, or just over three per minute. These include starts, stops, turns, throw-ins, and incidental contact with another player.

They found that the women who played soccer improved core stability in two crucial ways: First, their reaction time improved by 15 percent, which is to say that their muscles and nerves got better at stopping upper-body movement once it had begun. Second, the actual movement of the trunk decreased by 24 percent per incident.

The women assigned to the running group didn't improve in either measurement.

It's just one study, and it comes from a research group that seems unusually invested in showing that recreational soccer is a better form of exercise than steady-state running. Their studies don't show that running is worthless; the runners lost fat and improved in a variety of health measures. But the soccer players did measurably better in the same amount of time.

The big point is that you'll get more out of playing sports than you will from linear, steady-pace activities. Anything that involves unpredictable challenges and sudden changes in speed and direction will improve conditioning, core stability, hand-eye coordination, and overall athleticism. You won't get bigger and stronger, if that's your goal, but you will develop the ability to apply the strength and power you develop in the weight room.

I'm continually surprised to discover things I can do as an adult that I couldn't in my youth. In my mid-thirties a friend asked me to join his company's slow-pitch softball team. I'd been working out steadily for two decades by that point, but I was still amazed when I belted a line drive that went between the outfielders and rolled far enough for me to circle the bases with time to spare. It was the first home run I'd ever hit in my life.

Having said all this, I don't mean to imply that you *have* to get out and play an organized sport to get the benefits of the NROL for Abs program. Any physical activity will work. Nor am I saying that sports are risk-free. The more benefits they offer, the greater the chance for injury.

So let's look at your outside-the-gym options, and how to fit them into a structured training program.

THE HIERARCHY OF RISK AND REWARD

I've said throughout this book that all movement is good, and I'm sticking with it. But when you do two or three of Alwyn's workouts per week, your body is constantly in a state of recovery and repair. You have to be careful with the amount and type of stress you add to the stimulus of challenging and exhausting workouts.

Type of stress	Level of stress	Recommended recovery time
Muscular fatigue (prime movers)	High	2 days
Muscular fatigue (stabilizing muscles)	Medium	1 day
Joint/connective tissue fatigue	Medium	1 day
Energy-systems fatigue: Phase One Phase Two Phase Three	Low Moderate High	Less than 1 day 1 day 2 days
Neural fatigue: Phase One Phase Two Phase Three	Moderate High Very high	1 day 2 days 2–3 days

Let's start by looking at those workouts, and then figure out the best ways to complement them with other types of physical activity.

I use "energy-systems fatigue"—a nonscientific term I'm pretty sure I just made up—to estimate how deeply the workouts will tap into your energy supplies. Your body has three energy systems. The aerobic system, which your body uses throughout the day and night, uses a mix of fat and carbohydrate to keep your heart and lungs working and allow non-strenuous movement. The other two energy systems are anaerobic; your body uses them for short-term, relatively intense activities in which the primary source of fuel is carbohydrate. So if your muscles are depleted of some of their glycogen from your workout—strength training and metabolic work are both anaerobic activities—you don't want to go out a few hours later and do something that uses the same energy systems.

"Neural fatigue" is a real phenomenon, describing a state of emotional exhaustion that transcends whatever physical stress you're coping with. Let's say you're a competitive soccer player on a club team. A tough two-hour practice might exhaust your leg muscles, put stress on your joints, and induce energy-systems fatigue. But it wouldn't leave you emotionally drained. Conversely, a championship game would drain you physically and mentally. Your muscles would recover in two or three days, but it might take a week or two before your brain would be ready to compete again at that high a level.

The chart on page 245 lists some common recreational activities, and my best guess at how they affect all these variables.

You probably could go out and jog or play a mildly challenging sport a few hours after doing a Phase One workout. A yoga class would be no problem, unless it's a particularly intense style like Ashtanga (aka power yoga). In Phase Two, I recommend waiting until the next day before attempting an activity that requires a lot of fuel. Basketball, for example, uses the same energy systems as strength training, on top of the fact it beats the hell out of your lower-body joints and connective tissues.

So how do you use this information? Here's my take on the hierarchy of physical activities, from least to most demanding:

Do Anytime

These activities produce very little physical stress and require little or no recovery:

Golf (9 holes)

Informal sports-skills practice (shooting baskets, playing catch, hitting tennis balls, etc.)

Activity	MF(PM)	MF(SM)	J/CTF	ESF	NF
Baseball/softball	low	low	low to moderate	low	depends on length of game
Basketball	moderate	moderate	high	moderate to high	low
Bicycling	depends on distance	low	low	depends on distance	low
Golf	low	moderate	low	low	low
Hockey	moderate	moderate	high	high	low to moderate
Interval training (sprints, sled drags, etc.)	moderate	low to moderate	high	moderate to high	moderate to high
Martial arts (includes boxing and wrestling)	moderate to high	moderate to high	high	moderate to high	moderate to high (especially when sparring)
Running, short distance	low to moderate	low	moderate	low to moderate	low
Running, medium distance	moderate	moderate	moderate to high	moderate to high	low to moderate
Running, long distance	high	moderate	high	high	moderate to high
Soccer	moderate	low to moderate	moderate to high	moderate to high	low to moderate
Swimming	low	low to moderate	low	depends on distance	low to moderate
Tennis	low	low	moderate to high	depends on length of match	low to moderate
Walking	low	low	low	low	low
Yoga	low	moderate	low to moderate	low	low

Key:

MF(PM) = muscular fatigue (prime movers)

MF(SM) = muscular fatigue (stabilizing muscles)

J/CTF = joint/connective tissue fatigue

ESF = energy-systems fatigue

NF = neural fatigue

Walking or cycling, easy pace

Yoga (gentle styles)

Do on Non-Lifting Days

These sports and exercise choices are more fatiguing (yes, golf can be a workout for your lower back) and require recovery:

Golf (18 holes)

Martial arts (non-contact, for fitness or skill development)

Pick-up or recreational sports (baseball or softball, basketball, hockey, soccer, tennis)

Pilates or power yoga (Ashtanga)

Running, swimming, or cycling for fitness

Do with at Least a One-Day Break Before or After Lifting

These are the pursuits that take a toll on your body:

Competitive sports (basketball, hockey, soccer, tennis)

Interval training

Long-distance running, swimming, or cycling for performance

Martial arts (full contact)

If you do one of these on consecutive days with Alwyn's workouts, you want at least a day of rest at both ends. For example, if you go for a two-hour run on Sunday and lift weights on Monday, you want to make sure you don't do anything strenuous on Saturday and Tuesday.

Another example: Let's say you play basketball, hockey, or soccer in a competitive adult league on Tuesday nights. And let's say, like many of us, you like to hit the weight room on Monday, Wednesday, and Friday. Something has to give. Shifting to a Monday-Thursday-Saturday schedule would give you more recovery time and less risk of injury or burnout.

More simply: two days hard, one day light.

18

Answering the Questions You Haven't Yet Asked

ALWYN'S NROL for Abs program has these elements:

1. Dynamic warm-up
2. Core training
3. Strength training
3a. Power training (in Phase Three)
4. Metabolic training (in Phase Two and Phase Three)
5. Something else. It doesn't matter what it is, as long as it gets you up and moving and keeps you away from your computer, cell phone, and TV. It can be in or out of the gym. It can be as simple as walking or as complex as heli-skiing. We'd like you to do this almost every day of the week, including the days you lift.

There's also an unofficial sixth category: recovery. This includes foam rolling and flexibility exercises, either as part of your workout or completely separate from it.

Although there's no formal NROL for Abs diet, most of us get the best results from these nutritional practices:

1. Eat four to six meals and snacks a day.
2. Almost all of these should include protein. If you don't have protein, you should have something like an apple, which will leave you satisfied for a relatively long time.
3. Always have a pre- and/or post-workout shake. The closer to your workout, the better. If not a shake, then have milk, eggs, or something else that gets protein to your muscles with the least possible delay.
4. Eat breakfast.
5. Make simple changes first: Clean the junk food out of your diet, avoid liquid calories except for pre- and post-workout drinks, use alcohol judiciously, replace processed food with higher-protein and higher-fiber choices.
6. Don't cut calories until you've done Alwyn's workouts for at least four weeks. Then decide if you really need to create a larger calorie deficit.

Of course, if the workouts and diet recommendations were really that simple, this book would be a lot shorter than it is. And experience tells me that no matter how long a book is, readers will have an inexhaustible list of questions. To save time for both of us, I'll try to answer the ones I'm pretty sure someone will ask.

✳ **"I don't understand the workout charts."**
No matter how hard I work to explain the programs, it's still gibberish to a subset of readers. Happens every time. The only way to ensure that everyone understands everything on first glance is to use programs that are so simple no one could possibly be confused. But I'd have to find a new coauthor, because Alwyn doesn't dumb down his programs.

If you see something you don't understand, go to forums.jpfitness.com, and find the link to the dedicated discussion forum for *NROL for Abs*. Chances are, someone has already asked your question, and it's already been answered. Even if you happen to be first with a question, it'll probably be answered within a few hours.

✳ **"Is it okay if I do X instead of Y?"**
It's your body, your workout, your life. If you have a compelling reason to change something, it's your call. I rarely do a program exactly as it's written, including these. I'll give you a specific example:

When I started Phase Two, I quickly realized that I couldn't do the metabolic training after lifting. As soon as I pick up weights, I push myself to exhaustion, and

I'm not worth a damn at anything else I try to do. So I started doing my metabolic work before lifting, and that worked somewhat better. (My performance, I'll admit, was still disappointing.)

Alwyn has experimented with something similar: combining the dynamic warm-up and metabolic training at the front end of the workout, rather than splitting them up.

Does that mean you should experiment? Not unless you have a truly compelling reason. Alwyn knows that the system you see in *NROL for Abs* has worked for his clients. He might figure out something better in the near future, if he hasn't already, but that doesn't mean you'll have the same success tinkering with your own workouts. You might, or you might not. It depends on your knowledge of training in general and of your own body in particular.

I know what you're thinking: "I know my own body better than someone who's never worked with me one-on-one."

Of course you're right. But just because you know what your body *likes* to do doesn't mean you know what your body *needs* to do. This is a lesson I've learned and relearned countless times. My self-designed workouts inevitably default to the exercises and techniques that help me get where I am at the time I do them. If the goal is to progress beyond the development you've already attained, you need to try something you haven't yet done. Tinkering with it, more often than not, means you're selecting comfort and familiarity over results.

✳ **"Is there really no reason to do sit-ups and crunches? Like, ever?"**
Let's say you're a bodybuilder, or a model, or someone else who's extremely lean and needs or just wants to have abs with dramatic contours and separations. You need exercises that offer a hypertrophy stimulus. For that, Alwyn recommends crunches or weighted crunches on a Swiss ball. You're isolating the rectus abdominis as much as possible (although the obliques will always contribute to spinal flexion), you're extending the range of motion beyond what you can do with basic crunches on the floor, and you're not putting your lower back at extreme risk.

If you're an athlete in football, wrestling, or mixed martial arts, and you need to train spinal flexion for your sport, the overhead medicine-ball slam shown on page 170 is a great choice. You can also consider straight-leg sit-ups, either with your feet close together or spread apart. There's a lot of hip-flexor involvement in those movements, but that's a feature, not a bug. An MMA fighter who's trying to take down an opponent with a standing clinch needs to recruit every muscle involved in bending his torso forward against resistance.

For everyone else, I think you'll be very pleased with the results you get from the exercises Alwyn chose for this program.

✳ **"There aren't any biceps or triceps exercises in the program.
What am I supposed to do for my arms?"**

You're right. There aren't any exercises that specifically and exclusively target biceps, triceps, or forearms. Nor do any of them isolate your calves.

You will, however, work all those muscles. Chin-ups work your biceps through a full range of motion. Shoulder and chest presses hit your triceps. Deadlifts and rows with heavy weights build your forearms. And Alwyn's lower-body exercises will do a number on your calves, especially if, like me, your balance leaves a bit to be desired.

Would you build bigger arms if you did curls and extensions in addition to these exercises? Probably. Would the gains be measurable and noticeable? Possibly.

Alwyn has two big reasons for not including arm-isolating exercises:

1. These are demanding workouts. They affect your body systemically, and require systemic recovery. If you add an additional type of stress—particularly asymmetric stress, focused on specific muscles and joints—you've changed the recovery timetable. Now you're in uncharted territory. Alwyn didn't design these workouts with muscle- or joint-specific recovery in mind.

2. The two most important goals of the program are to develop core stability, endurance, and strength, in conjunction with improved body composition (more muscle, less fat). Secondary goals include better conditioning and athleticism. Additional arm exercises don't help you reach any of those goals. They don't work your core, make you leaner, or help you become a better athlete.

Frankly, I'll be surprised if you get to the end of Phase Three, look in the mirror, and tell yourself the program would've worked better with curls and extensions.

✳ **"I'm embarrassed to admit this, but I can't do this much exercise
in a single workout. What happens if I split it up?"**

This is one circumstance in which you have to trust what your body is telling you. In this case, it's crying "uncle." Here's how Alwyn would split it up:

1. Lift weights two times a week (Monday-Thursday, say, or Tuesday-Friday).
2. Do the metabolic work on separate days.

3. Do light physical activity, even if it's just stretching and foam rolling, on two other days.

A one-week schedule might look like this:

Monday	Tuesday	Wednesday	Thursday	Friday	Saturday	Sunday
Weights	Metabolic work	Light exercise	Weights	Metabolic work	Light exercise	Off

✳   **"What should I do after I finish Phase Three? Can I go back and repeat the program? If so, should I change anything?"**

This is probably the most important question of all, and I've saved it for last. Short answer: Absolutely you can repeat the program. When you go through it a second time, you'll be stronger and better conditioned, with improved mobility and athleticism. Even if you do the exact same workouts the exact same way, it's not the same you who's doing them. You'll be able to work harder in multiple ways:

- choose more challenging variations of exercises
- work with heavier weights
- do more sets of the strength exercises, and push yourself further on the metabolic work

Another option is to repeat the workout structure with different exercises. Let's start with core training. We show so many stabilization exercises that you could repeat Phase One at least twice without duplicating your exercise choices. With a bit of sleuthing you can find new dynamic- and integrated-stabilization exercises to slot in when you repeat Phase Two and Phase Three.

Remember that there's no such thing as a magic exercise, and once you've done the program exactly as Alwyn designed it, you can try it again with exercises of your own choosing. As long as you stick to the same basic movement patterns—a squat for a squat, a press for a press, a row for a row—the choices are nearly unlimited.

Another way to approach the workouts the second or third time through is to use heavier weights with lower reps in Phase One and Phase Two, and lighter weights with higher reps in Phase Three. And remember that Phase Two has an optional component called Maximum Strength. If you didn't use it the first time through, you can always circle back and try it the second or third time you do the program.

19

The End of
the Beginning

I AM A TRUE BELIEVER. I truly believe in the power of exercise to transform not just the body you see in the mirror or measure on a scale, but the attitude that shapes how you perceive that body. An exerciser, a lifter, realizes that he or she can do things that once seemed unlikely, if not impossible. Exercise teaches us to appreciate the plasticity of our bodies and brains. We learn that it's possible to reshape the former and reorient the latter.

Of course, there are limits on that plasticity, and this is hardly news to anyone who shares our mutually agreed upon concept of reality. I learned early enough in life that my 110-pound weight set from Sears, even when combined with the primitive Universal machine at my high school, wouldn't transform me from a skinny third-string football player into a hulking all-American.

What kept me interested in training, what made me passionate about it, wasn't the anticipation of future magic. It was the acquisition of solid, measurable gains in strength and size. I went from someone who got thrown around the football field like a chew toy to someone who could kinda-sorta hold his own, in deservedly limited playing time. Stardom was never in the cards, but thanks to the weights, I didn't have to settle for suckdom. Mediocrity was an achievement. I worked hard for it, even if it wasn't something I could put on my résumé.

Then there's the issue of appearance. As a skinny kid, a few pounds of muscle went a long way. Guys still mocked me—I vividly remember the relentless and borderline sadistic teasing I got from a locker-room attendant at the pool where I worked summers as a lifeguard—but girls seemed to appreciate it. My dating prospects improved dramatically each June, the start of swimsuit season, and returned to baseline in September. Unless my personality got better with daily sun exposure, it must've been the physique.

Don't get me wrong: My body was never anything to brag about. I was never the strongest or leanest or most muscular guy in the room. But thanks to training, I was no longer the *least* muscular. My incremental achievements in the weight room foreshadowed incremental achievements in other areas of my life. Once I stopped looking at the world in terms of its impediments, I discovered some of the paths over, around, and through them.

Which, at long last, brings me to my final point.

When Alwyn and I decided to write a book with "abs" in the title, we worried about making a promise we couldn't deliver to many of our readers. That's why we've invested so many words in describing the process of training and so few on the results of it, like the wonderful life that awaits the man or woman with single-digit body fat and abs like horizontal wind chimes.

Some of you have that already. Many will achieve it, thanks to Alwyn's workout system. But for others, it's an unrealistic expectation. What's possible for everyone is what I just described: the satisfaction of knowing that you now have something you didn't have a week or a month or a year ago. You're stronger, leaner, and more muscular than you would've been if you hadn't done these programs. Are you as lean and fit as you wanted to be? Maybe you are. Maybe you exceeded your expectations. Or maybe you realize you still have a way to go.

I don't know about you, but that describes every aspect of my life. Just in the short interval between *NROL* books, I changed the way I worked out so I could recover from injuries. I pushed myself far beyond my comfort zone to play one sport and coach another. I've taken risks professionally and tried to do the best for my family, even though, as every parent knows, the role of kids is to lower their parents' expectations for order in the universe.

For me, it's all a series of incremental steps forward, sideways, and occasionally backward. There are no moments of absolute success or failure. You succeed in a training program because of the accumulation of healthy meals and vigorous work-outs. Your program isn't ruined by one bad meal or one missed training session. It's not even set back in any significant way. It's just one day in which you didn't move forward.

Maximize the good days and minimize the others, and you will succeed.

Appendix

The Rules

These are the rules from all three *NROL* books, starting with the basic rules of exercise:

1. Do something.
2. Do something you like.
3. The rest is just details.

I can't see any reason to argue with myself here. As I wrote in the first book, "Exercise scientists don't agree on much, but I think they'd all acknowledge that the most important benefits of exercise accrue when someone goes from sedentary to moderately active."

You're more likely to stick with a fitness routine if it's based on something you enjoy doing. We can argue endlessly about which type of exercise is better or worse than others, but I think it's self-evident that you'll get more out of an activity you do consistently for life than something you give up on because it's not fun or convenient, or because it disrupts your work or family life.

These are the original New Rules of Lifting:

1. The best muscle-building exercises are the ones that use your muscles the way they're designed to work.
2. Exercises that use lots of muscles in coordinated action are better than those that force muscles to work in isolation.
3. To build size, you must build strength.
4. To build size and strength, you must train hard but infrequently, with plenty of recovery time between workouts.
5. The goal of each workout is to set a record.
6. The weight you lift is a tool to reach your goals. It is not a goal by itself.
7. Don't "do the machines."
8. A workout is only as good as the adaptations it produces.
9. There is no magic system of exercises, sets, and reps.
10. Don't judge a system by the physique of the person promoting it.
11. You'll get better results working your ass off on a bad program than you will loafing through a good program.
12. Fast lifting is not more dangerous than slow lifting.
13. A good warm-up doesn't have to make your body warm.
14. Stretching is not a warm-up.
15. You don't need to warm up to stretch.
16. Lifting by itself may increase your flexibility.
17. Aerobic fitness is not a matter of life and death.
18. You don't need to do endurance exercise to burn fat.
19. When you combine serious strength training with serious endurance exercise, your body will probably choose endurance over muscle and strength.
20. If it's not fun, you're doing something wrong.

These are the New Rules of Lifting for Women:

1. The purpose of lifting weights is to build muscle.
2. Muscle is hard to build.
3. Results come from hard work.
4. Hard work includes lifting heavier weights.
5. From time to time, you have to break some of the old rules.
6. No workout will make you taller.

7. Muscles in men and women are essentially identical.
8. Muscle strength is a matter of life and death.
9. A muscle's "pump" is not the same as muscle growth.
10. Endurance exercise is an option, not a necessity, for fat loss.
11. "Aerobics" doesn't mean what you think it means.
12. Calorie restriction is the worst idea ever.
13. Traditional weight-loss advice is fatally flawed.
14. To reach your goals, you may need to eat more.
15. On balance, a balanced-macro diet is best.
16. Protein is the queen of macronutrients.
17. More meals are better than fewer.
18. Don't do programs designed for someone else's needs.
19. You don't need to isolate small muscles to make them bigger and stronger.
20. Every exercise is a "core" exercise.
21. The biggest blocks to your success could be the ones you've erected.

Finally, the New Rules of Lifting for Abs:

1. The most important role of the abdominal muscles is to protect your spine.
2. You can't protect your spine by doing exercises that damage it.
3. The size of your abdominal muscles doesn't matter.
4. The appearance of your abs doesn't matter either.
5. The core includes all the muscles that attach to your hips, pelvis, and lower back.
6. The lats are part of the core.
7. The crunch is not a core exercise.
8. Your spine is already flexed, and flexing it more just makes it worse.
9. Stability in your lower back depends on mobility in the joints above and below it.
10. You can't out-exercise a hunger-inducing lifestyle.
11. Your computer is the enemy of your abs.
12. TV and video games are almost as bad as your computer.
13. You can sleep your way to a better body . . . or not sleep your way to a bigger belly.
14. "Convenience" food is designed for one reason: to make you eat more convenience food.
15. Processed food makes you stupid and depressed.
16. All that said, calories still matter more than anything else.
17. Don't do a complicated intervention until you've tried all the simple ones.

Notes

Introduction

Physical therapists: I refer to two physical therapists in this chapter. The one who worked on my shoulder is Bill Hartman, whom Alwyn has called "the smartest man in the fitness industry." Bill is co-owner, with Mike Robertson, of Indianapolis Fitness and Sports Training, and one of those guys who always seems to have a grasp of the most important new information and exercise techniques a year or two before the rest of us catch on. The second is Keith Scott (his website is at backtoformfitness.com), who worked the knots out of my right leg and gave me a corrective exercise program that allowed me to return to playing sports after months as a gimp.

Chapter 1

Stuart McGill: I've been strongly influenced by Dr. McGill's books *Low Back Disorders* and *Ultimate Back Fitness and Performance.* The quotes I used are from *LBD*, pp. 9–10. Both books are available at his website, backfitpro.com.

Injury prevention: Zazulak et al., "Neuromuscular control of trunk stability:

clinical implications for sports injury prevention." *Journal of the American Academy of Orthopaedic Surgeons* 2008; 16: 497–505. This review noted that, while deficits in core stability predicted knee injuries in female athletes, this wasn't true for the men. Only a prior history of lower-back pain predicted knee injuries for male athletes.

Size of muscles: Gibbons et al., "Isokinetic and psychophysical lifting strength, static back muscle endurance, and magnetic resonance imaging of the paraspinal muscles as predictors of low back pain in men." *Scandinavian Journal of Rehabilitation Medicine* 1997; 29 (3): 187–191. This study found "weak but significant correlations" between the size of spinal-erector muscles and frequency of lower-back pain in a sample of middle-aged men. Reduced muscle size is most likely a result of atrophy in the men with back pain, rather than a sign that building these muscles reduces the risk of pain. Normally, these muscles are resistant to atrophy with aging, which seems to indicate that maintaining their size is important to their function as spinal stabilizers. But I couldn't find any research showing that intentional hypertrophy of these muscles—making them bigger through targeted exercises—leads to improved spinal stability or a reduced risk of back pain.

Ab strength and longevity: Katzmarzyk and Craig, "Musculoskeletal fitness and risk of mortality." *Medicine & Science in Sports & Exercise* 2002; 34 (5): 740–744.

U.S. Army study: Childs et al., "Effects of sit-up training versus core stabilization exercises on sit-up performance." *Medicine & Science in Sports & Exercise* 2009; 41 (11): 2072–2083. I learned about this one via Patrick Ward's blog, optimumsportsperformance.com.

A potential confounder in this study is the fact that about two-thirds of the soldiers did sit-ups outside the formal training program. When I read that, my first instinct was to drop the whole thing. But the researchers, after admitting that this may have blurred the results, went on to note that there weren't any differences between the groups that did the extra sit-ups and those that didn't.

So I think the basic idea remains supportable: Exercises designed to enhance core stability do help you increase core endurance on an exercise you haven't actually practiced. I just wish there were more people in the study who hadn't practiced the exercise.

"like giant raviolis": This was an actual cover line from *Men's Fitness* magazine in 1991 or 1992. I started working there full-time in early '92, so I wasn't part of the creative team that can take credit for it.

Chapter 2

Neutral zone: Much of the information in this chapter comes from a pair of articles that appeared back to back in the April 2007 issue of *Strength and Conditioning Journal,* which is published by the National Strength and Conditioning Association: "Core Training: Stabilizing the Confusion," by Mark Faries and Mike Greenwood (p. 10), and "Lumbar Stabilization: An Evidence-Based Approach for the Athlete with Low-Back Pain," by Morey Kolber and Kristina Beekhuizen (p. 26). Both are review articles, citing more than one hundred individual studies altogether.

Gluteal amnesia: McGill, *Ultimate Back Fitness and Performance,* p. 148.

Ab slide versus crunch: Escamilla et al., "An electromyographic analysis of commercial and common abdominal exercises: implications for rehabilitation and training." *Journal of Orthopaedic & Sports Physical Therapy* 2006; 36 (2): 45–57. Youdas et al., "An electromyographic analysis of the ab-slide exercise, abdominal crunch, supine double leg thrust and side bridge in healthy young adults: implications for rehabilitation professionals." *Journal of Strength and Conditioning Research* 2008; 22 (6): 1939–1946.

Hip-flexor tests: Michael Boyle, *Advances in Functional Training* (On Target Publications, 2010), pp. 114–115.

Role of adductors and abductors: Activation of the gluteus medius during a standing single-leg exercise is shown in McGill et al., "Exercises for the torso performed in a standing posture: spine and hip motion and motor patterns and spine load." *Journal of Strength and Conditioning Research* 2009; 23 (2): 455–464.

Various roles of hip flexors and adductors are discussed in *Anatomy Trains,* by Thomas Myers (Churchill Livingstone, 2001).

Lats and glutes working together: This is also from *Anatomy Trains,* one of the most interesting and instructive books I've read about the structure and function of the human muscular system.

A lot of us think of muscles in isolation; that's why we do exercises that target our lats, abs, biceps, or whatever. Or maybe we think of them in groups according to the functions they perform. So the deltoids are connected to the pectorals because they work together when we do bench presses. But that's not the only way muscles work together. They also transfer force from one to the other, even if they aren't contiguously linked. That's how the lats and glutes on opposite sides of your body work together; Myers calls it the "back functional line." Another example: The front functional line transfers force from the left pectoralis major (chest muscle) to the left rectus abdominis, and then over to the adductor muscles on the inner thigh of the right leg.

Most of the book is based on painstaking examination of human cadavers, which is how scientists uncovered the secrets of our fascia, the connective tissues that link muscles to one another in ways that are impossible to see from the outside. Especially surprising is the line of fascia that links the bottoms of our feet to the front of our scalp. Myers calls it the "superficial back line."

I wouldn't go as far as to say that the pectorals have a role in stabilizing your core—if you don't draw the line somewhere, you'd have to include all 640 human muscles, including those in your eyes and ears. But Alwyn and I think it's perfectly legitimate and accurate to include the lats, glutes, adductors, and abductors in the conversation.

Core muscle activation during deadlift: Juker et al., "Quantitative intramuscular myoelectric activity of lumbar portions of psoas and the abdominal wall during a wide variety of tasks." *Medicine & Science in Sports & Exercise* 1998; 30 (2): 301–310.

The McBride material is available online at strengthcoach.com/mcbride-new-training-techniques.pdf.

Along with colleagues at Appalachian State, McBride published a study that compared squats and deadlifts to three isometric exercises performed on a Swiss ball: Nuzzo et al., "Trunk muscle activity during stability ball and free weight exercises." *Journal of Strength and Conditioning Research* 2008; 22 (1): 95–102. This study looks only at the activity of back-extensor muscles, without measuring abdominal muscle activation.

Chapter 3

Functions of abdominal muscles: Personal Trainer Manual, 2nd ed. pp. 54–58. Published by the American Council on Exercise, 1996.

Defensive posture: Anatomy Trains, p. 118.

Walking upright to conserve energy: Sockol et al., "Chimpanzee locomotor energetics and the origin of human bipedalism." *Proceedings of the National Academy of Sciences* 2007; 104 (30): 12265–12269. I found this reference in "Walking on Two Feet Was an Energy-Saving Step," by Roxanne Khamsi in the July 16, 2007, issue of *New Scientist.*

MMA clinch: Thanks to Chad Waterbury for explaining to me how and why he uses spinal-flexion exercises to train mixed-martial-arts fighters.

Soreness: Soreness isn't necessarily a sign that muscles are growing faster than they do when they're not sore. It's just a pretty good way for lifelong gym rats like me to tell that I've forced the muscles in question to do something they weren't expecting. I never try to make myself sore, and don't recommend that anyone else should seek soreness either. I just notice it when it happens.

Muscle activation in single versus multiple planes of movement: McGill et al., "Exercises for the torso performed in a standing posture: spine and hip motion and motor patterns and spine load." *Journal of Strength and Conditioning Research* 2009; 23 (2): 455–464. In this study, McGill and his colleagues tested a series of "functional" exercises—several of which appear in Alwyn's workouts—and found that most of them resulted in low levels of muscle activation, despite the fact the male college students who performed the exercises found them extremely difficult and strenuous.

The one exception was the hand walkout on the floor. (You get into a push-up position and walk your hands out as far as you can while keeping your lumbar spine in a neutral position.) The *average* activation of the rectus abdominis muscle was 100 percent. In the Discussion section of the study, the researchers suggested that maximum muscle activation was possible because all the movement stayed in a single plane. When your body has to work in multiple planes of motion, the effort it takes to keep your spine in its neutral zone prevents muscles from working at full capacity.

The take-away message is what I wrote in Chapter 3: If you want to work muscles as hard as possible to develop size and strength, choose the most straightforward, single-plane exercises. If you want to work your *body* as hard as possible, in a systemic way, you should probably choose exercises that involve multiple planes of motion. That brings more muscles into play, even if fewer muscles are working as hard as they possibly can.

Obviously, the best workout program would involve both types of exercises— the multiplane exercises to develop coordination and core stability, and to make the workouts more effective in terms of total energy cost; and the single-plane exercises for maximum strength and mass development.

Chapter 6

Pavel Tsatsouline: Pavel, who immigrated to the United States from Russia, is best-known today for introducing and popularizing kettlebells in his new country. But before I'd heard of kettlebells, I absorbed Pavel's ideas about strength training and conditioning in books like *Power to the People!* (Dragon Door, 1999) and *Bullet-proof Abs* (2000), the latter a sequel to *Beyond Crunches* (1998).

He was one of the first fitness gurus I met who expressed open disdain for muscle-isolating exercises in general, and crunches in particular. Pavel (no one refers to him by his last name) talked about building muscle and strength by doing low-rep sets with near-max weights at a time when "3 sets of 10" was the default setting for most lifters.

I can't say for sure that *Beyond Crunches* and *Bullet-proof Abs* brought the ab wheel back from obscurity. Strength coaches and trainers don't work in isolation; they share and fine-tune ideas for years before they emerge as hot new trends in health clubs. But I can say with near certainty that I hadn't considered doing the ab-wheel rollout before I saw it in Pavel's books.

Chapter 9

Mobility-stability continuum: Advances in Functional Training, pp. 31–33. Boyle credits physical therapist Gray Cook with first explaining this concept to him. Cook is the author of *Athletic Body in Balance* (Human Kinetics, 2003).

Chapter 13

Average person heavier: "XXXL: Why Are We So Fat?" by Elizabeth Kolbert. *The New Yorker*, July 20, 2009, pp. 73–77.

Total calories available per day: USDA/Economic Research Service, updated February 27, 2009.

Weight loss with exercise: King et al., "Individual variability following 12 weeks of supervised exercise: identification and characterization of compensation for exercise-induced weight loss." *International Journal of Obesity* 2008; 32 (1): 177–184.

University of Washington study: McCann et al., "Changes in plasma lipids and dietary intake accompanying shifts in perceived workload and stress." *Psychosomatic Medicine* 1990; 52: 97–108.

Laval University study: Chaput et al., "Glycemic instability and spontaneous energy intake: association with knowledge-based work." *Psychosomatic Medicine* 2008; 70: 797–804.

This study involved fourteen young, normal-weight women, so we can't make too much of the results. I just thought it was interesting that this experiment, which references the aforementioned University of Washington study while cleaning up some of its loose ends, came up with a similar number for the excess calorie consumption triggered by knowledge-based work. The first study, relying on food diaries, counted 240 excess calories per day, while this one, using precise knowledge of the food consumed, found that the study subjects ate 253 extra calories immediately after forty-five minutes of an intentionally stressful computer test.

Whether the numbers will change with a more diverse group of study subjects is TBD; the Laval researchers are in the process of finding out.

"Brain Candy": The information in this sidebar came from more sources than I could list. It's mostly textbook stuff.

Appetite control and knowledge-based work: Chaput and Tremblay, "The glucostatic theory of appetite control and the risk of obesity and diabetes." *International Journal of Obesity* 2009; 33: 46–53.

TV time and waist size: Healy et al., "Television time and continuous metabolic risk in physically active adults." *Medicine & Science in Sports & Exercise* 2008; 40(4): 639–645. I found analysis of the study in an article by Scott Riewald called "Nothing Bad Can Happen Sitting in Front of the TV. Right?" It ran in the June 2009 issue of *Strength and Conditioning Journal.*

Video games and health markers: Weaver et al., "Health-risk correlates of video-game playing among adults." *American Journal of Preventive Medicine* 2009; 37(4): 379–380.

Sleep and body fat: Van Cauter and Knutson, "Sleep and the epidemic of obesity in children and adults." *European Journal of Endocrinology* 2008; 159: S59–S66. Also the Chaput and Tremblay paper mentioned earlier.

Increased hunger: Spiegel et al., "Sleep curtailment in healthy young men is associated with decreased leptin levels, elevated ghrelin levels and increased hunger and appetite." *Annals of Internal Medicine* 2004; 141: 846–850. (This study was summarized in the Van Cauter and Knutson paper cited above.)

Ghrelin is a hunger-inducing hormone, produced in the stomach. It's the yin to leptin's yang; when it rises, you get hungry. I didn't use the study's information about ghrelin because I was following the rule of threes. If I couldn't make my points about the danger of sleep deficits with my once-over-lightly explanations of cortisol, leptin, and insulin, it's unlikely that adding a fourth hormone to the section would fix the problem.

This sleep-deficit study used young men as its subjects, so the results might have been different with women or with older subjects of either gender. The Van Cauter and Knutson paper reports that "the impact of short sleep on obesity risk appears greater in children than adults, and greater in young adulthood than in midlife or late life."

I don't know about you, but I'm encouraged by this finding. I was a big sleeper in my youth—early to bed, early to rise, dead to the world in between—but in middle age I find that ridiculously insignificant problems can keep me tossing and turning for hours. It doesn't seem to affect my appetite in any noticeable way.

Sedentary time and waist size: Healy et al., "Objectively measured sedentary time, physical activity, and metabolic risk." *Diabetes Care* 2008; 31: 369–371.

Taking more breaks: Healy et al., "Breaks in sedentary time." *Diabetes Care* 2008; 31: 661–666.

Weight gain leads to less walking: Levine et al., "The role of free-living daily walking in human weight gain and obesity." *Diabetes* 2008; 57: 548–554. James Levine and colleagues are the Mayo Clinic researchers referred to in the next section.

Dog walking: "The Best Walking Partner: Man vs. Dog" by Tara Parker-Pope, *New York Times* online, December 14, 2009.

Factors in disrupted sleep habits: Many of these are from "How to Get Great Sleep," by Hara Estroff Marano, from the November 2003 issue of *Psychology Today*.

Chapter 14

Food is cheaper today: This is from the *New Yorker* article cited earlier.

Parallels between food and tobacco industries: The End of Overeating, by David A. Kessler, M.D. (Rodale, 2009). The explicit comparison of food and tobacco marketing is on p. 240, but in this section I've encapsulated information from throughout the book.

Genes and obesity: Li et al., "Cumulative effects and predictive value of common obesity-susceptibility variants identified by genome-wide association studies." *American Journal of Clinical Nutrition* 2010; 91 (1): 184–190.

I won't claim to be a serious student of human genetics. Common sense tells us that human body weight and adiposity are to some extent genetic traits, like height and hair color. Your kids probably have the same shape you had at their ages. Now that you're an adult, though, chances are your shape reflects a combination of your parents' profile and your lifestyle choices. You might be bigger or smaller. You understand you have some control of your weight and fitness profile. Common sense, right?

The study I cite here, which looks at a dozen gene variants associated with obesity, concludes that "their predictive value for obesity risk is limited." That doesn't mean the risk is nonexistent, just that genes are only part of the story.

HFCS: John S. White, "Misconceptions about high-fructose corn syrup: is it uniquely responsible for obesity, reactive dicarbonyl compounds, and advanced glycation endproducts?" *The Journal of Nutrition* 2009; 139: 1219S–1227S.

Dr. White is a consultant to the food industry, so there's the obvious potential for bias in his conclusion that "HFCS does not pose a unique dietary risk in healthy individuals or diabetics." I confess that I used this paper because it rounds up a lot of research that would've taken me hours to compile on my own. The evidence, in my view, doesn't exonerate the food industry; it simply shows that HFCS is part of a much bigger and more systemic problem with our current food chain.

Processed food and mental health: Akbaraly et al., "Dietary pattern and depressive symptoms in middle age." *British Journal of Psychiatry* 2009; 195 (5): 408–413. Akbaraly et al., "Education attenuates the association between dietary patterns and cognition." *Dementia and Geriatric Cognitive Disorders* 2009; 27 (2): 147–154.

Utilitarian view of food: *The Body Fat Solution,* by Tom Venuto (Avery, 2009), pp. 83–84.

Chapter 15

Water content of body: John D. Kirschmann and Nutrition Search, Inc., *Nutrition Almanac,* 6th ed. (McGraw-Hill, 2007), p. 85.

Low-fat diet and estrogen: Gann et al., "The effects of a low-fat/high-fiber diet on sex hormone levels and menstrual cycling in premenopausal women: a 12-month randomized trial (the diet and hormone study)." *Cancer* 2003; 98 (9); 1870–1879.

Minimum requirements of protein, fat, and carbs: Dietary reference intakes for energy, carbohydrate, fiber, fat, fatty acids, cholesterol, protein, and amino acids (The National Academies Press, 2005). You can read the entire book online at books.nap.edu.

Protein consensus: Wilson and Wilson, "Contemporary issues in protein requirements and consumption for resistance trained athletes." *Journal of the International Society of Sports Nutrition* 2006; 3 (1): 7–27. This is a terrific roundup of protein research, if you're curious about the subject and looking for a one-stop resource.

Three major protein benefits: Paddon-Jones et al., "Protein, weight management, and satiety." *American Journal of Clinical Nutrition* 2008; 87 (supplement): 1558S–

1561S. This paper was presented at a conference called Protein Summit 2007: Exploring the Impact of High-Quality Protein on Optimal Health, and was sponsored by food-industry groups including the National Dairy Council, National Pork Board, Egg Nutrition Center, and National Cattlemen's Beef Association.

As with the HFCS paper I cited earlier, I could've supported the exact same conclusions about protein with studies that weren't sponsored or supported by the major beneficiaries of their conclusions. The three major claims, as far as I know, aren't controversial. I've seen them made often, in countless peer-reviewed studies. As before, this review just happened to have everything I was looking for in one convenient location.

Protein increases muscle mass: Robert Wolfe, "Skeletal muscle protein metabolism and resistance exercise." *Journal of Nutrition* 2006; 136: 525S–528S.

Thermic effect of carbs and fat: Eric Jequier, "Is fat intake a risk factor for fat gain in children?" *Journal of Clinical Endocrinology & Metabolism* 2001; 86 (3): 980–983.

Minimal protein reduces thigh circumference: Campbell et al., "The recommended dietary allowance for protein may not be adequate for older people to maintain skeletal muscle." *The Journals of Gerontology Series A, Biological Sciences and Medical Sciences* 2001; 56 (6): M373–M380.

Thigh circumference and longevity: Heitmann and Frederiksen, "Thigh circumference and risk of heart disease and premature death: prospective cohort study." *British Medical Journal* 2009; 339: b3292.

Protein in foods: I used a combination of *Nutrition Almanac* and the USDA database. The two sources list things in different ways, so with some foods I just had to pick the one that seemed more typical of the way you and I measure food.

Dietary fat and heart disease: Oh et al., "Dietary fat intake and risk of coronary heart disease in women: 20 years of follow-up of the Nurses' Health Study." *American Journal of Epidemiology* 2005; 161 (7): 672–679.

U.S. government advocates more corn production: Greg Critser, *Fat Land* (Houghton Mifflin, 2003). More recent books, including the aforementioned *The End of Overeating*, by Dr. David Kessler, and the not-yet-cited *The Omnivore's Dilemma* (Penguin, 2006) and *In Defense of Food* (Penguin, 2008), both by Michael Pollan, lay out the same sequence of events, more or less. However, Critser's book was the first I read in this new genre of how-we-got-so-fat books, and I gladly mention it whenever I get a chance.

The Pollan books are brilliant—I defy anyone to read three pages of either book at random and not come away feeling smarter—but you can't beat Critser's *Fat Land* for its combination of depth, analysis, and witty presentation.

Diet comparisons: Gardner et al., "Comparison of the Atkins, Zone, Ornish, and LEARN diets for change in weight and related risk factors among overweight premenopausal women." *Journal of the American Medical Association* 2007; 297 (9): 969–977.

You can find Gardner's YouTube video "The Battle of the Diets: Is Anyone Winning (at Losing)?" here: youtube.com/watch?v=eREuZEdMAVo. I've watched it twice, and I recommend it wholeheartedly to anyone who is willing to invest an hour and a quarter to listen to a breezy, audience-friendly overview not just of how and why diets work or don't work, but also how hard it is to study diets.

Cooking and evolution: Elizabeth Pennisi, "Did cooked tubers spur the evolution of big brains?" *Science* 1999; 283: 2004–2005. Katherine Harmon, "Humans feasting on grains for at least 100,000 years." *Scientific American* Observations blog, December 17, 2009.

History of agriculture: In *The Omnivore's Dilemma,* p. 129, Michael Pollan asserts that the grasses themselves—the wild progenitors of wheat, rice, and corn—spontaneously evolved from perennials into hardy annuals, the seeds of which became irresistibly appealing to Neolithic humans.

Human stature and inequality: Burkhard Bilger, "The Height Gap." *The New Yorker,* April 4, 2005.

Glycemic load: Frank Hu, "Diet and cardiovascular disease prevention: the need for a paradigm shift." *Journal of the American College of Cardiology* 2007; 50 (1); 22–24.

Charts comparing glycemic, insulin, and satiety measures: I got the idea to compare all these indices from my friend Alan Aragon's self-published book, *Girth Control* (alanaragon.com). I ended up pulling numbers from a variety of sources, none of which agree with each other across the board. I found the insulin and satiety indices from David Mendosa's terrific website, mendosa.com. My comparisons of glycemic index and glycemic load started with p. 15 in *Nutrition Almanac,* but when I tried to compare those numbers to Alan's and to lists I found on the Mendosa site, I gave myself a massive headache. Sometimes each source for GI and GL was different from the others. I'm sure the numbers I use are in the right ballpark, but they might be off by a point or two from some of the compilations that are currently available.

Constipation: Inner Hygiene: Constipation and the Pursuit of Health in Modern

Society (Oxford University Press, 2000), by James C. Whorton, p. 6. I accessed this quote via Amazon.com's "look inside" feature.

Machine processing of wheat: Pollan, *In Defense of Food*, p. 105.

Bernarr Macfadden: Mr. America (Harper, 2009), by Mark Adams, p. 162.

Rise of trans fats: This information comes from a variety of sources—including, I confess, Wikipedia, which is where I got the Crisco chronology. The rise of margarine is detailed in *In Defense of Food*, pp. 32–36. Other info about the chemical structure of all fats, including trans fat, came from *Nutrition Almanac*. The timeline for CSPI's campaign to get fast-food restaurants to use trans fats is from "The Tragic Legacy of Center for Science in the Public Interest," by Mary G. Enig (westonaprice.org, January 6, 2003).

Dietary fat and weight: Forouhi et al., "Dietary fat intake and subsequent weight change in adults: results from the European Prospective Investigation into Cancer and Nutrition cohorts." *American Journal of Clinical Nutrition* 2009; 90 (6): 1632–1641.

Fat metabolism: DeLany et al., "Differential oxidation of individual fatty acids in humans." *American Journal of Clinical Nutrition* 2000; 72: 905–911.

Dangers of fat imbalance: Kiecolt-Glaser et al., "Depressive symptoms, omega-6: omega-3 fatty acids, and inflammation in older adults." *Psychosomatic Medicine* 2007; 69: 217–224.

Chapter 16

Milk and muscle gains: Josse et al., "Body composition and strength changes in women with milk and resistance exercise." *Medicine & Science in Sports & Exercise* 2009, epub. Hartman et al., "Consumption of fat-free fluid milk after resistance exercise promotes greater lean mass accretion than does consumption of soy or carbohydrate in young, novice, male weightlifters." *American Journal of Clinical Nutrition* 2007; 86 (2): 373–381.

Breakfast: Malinauskas et al., "Dieting practices, weight perceptions, and body composition: A comparison of normal weight, overweight, and obese college females." *Nutrition Journal* 2006; 5:11.

Normal weight, overweight, obese: These categories are determined by body-mass index. You can calculate your own at nhlbisupport.com/bmi/bmicalc.htm.

Meal frequency: Duval et al., "Physical activity is a confounding factor of the relation between eating frequency and body composition." *American Journal of Clinical Nutrition* 2008; 88: 1200–1205.

Pre- vs. post-workout protein: Tipton et al., "Timing of amino acid-carbohydrate ingestion alters anabolic response of muscle to resistance exercise." *American Journal of Physiology: Endocrinology and Metabolism* 2001; 281: E197–E206. Tipton et al., "Stimulation of net muscle protein synthesis by whey protein ingestion before and after exercise." *American Journal of Physiology: Endocrinology and Metabolism* 2007; 292: E71–E76. Fujita et al., "Essential amino acid and carbohydrate ingestion before resistance exercise does not enhance postexercise muscle protein synthesis." *Journal of Applied Physiology* 2009; 106: 1730–1739.

Milk protein: Lacroix et al., "Compared with casein or total milk protein, digestion of milk soluble proteins is too rapid to sustain the anabolic postprandial amino acid requirement." *American Journal of Clinical Nutrition* 2006; 84 (5): 1070–1079.

Weighing yourself: Van Wormer et al., "The impact of regular self-weighing on weight management: a systematic literature review." *International Journal of Behavioral Nutrition and Physical Activity* 2008; 5: 54–63. Hat tip to our friend Mike Roussell (nakednutritionnetwork.com), who sent this study to me while I was writing the nutrition chapters. Mike is a Ph.D. candidate at Penn State University who has a self-published book, *Your Naked Nutrition Guide*, and has contributed chapters to several books.

Carb cycling: I cribbed the basics from "A Beginner's Guide to Carb Cycling," by Matt McGorry, which I edited during the year in which I worked at tmuscle.com. The article was posted on April 15, 2009.

Drinking habits: Tolstrup et al., "Alcohol drinking frequency in relation to subsequent changes in waist circumference." *American Journal of Clinical Nutrition* 2008; 87: 957–963. I also referred to "A Musclehead's Guide to Alcohol," by Alan Aragon, another article I edited at tmuscle.com. It was posted on September 17, 2008.

Chapter 17

Core stability and sports: Pedersen et al., "Recreational soccer can improve the reflex response to sudden trunk loading among untrained women." *Journal of Strength and Conditioning Research* 2009; 23 (9): 2621–2626.

Soccer versus running: Krustrup et al., "Recreational soccer is an effective health-promoting activity for untrained men." *British Journal of Sports Medicine* 2009; 43 (11): 825–831.

Index

MORE TITLES IN THE
NEW RULES OF LIFTING SERIES

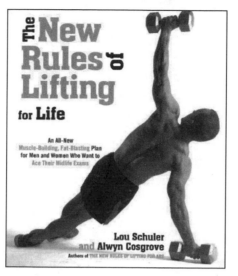
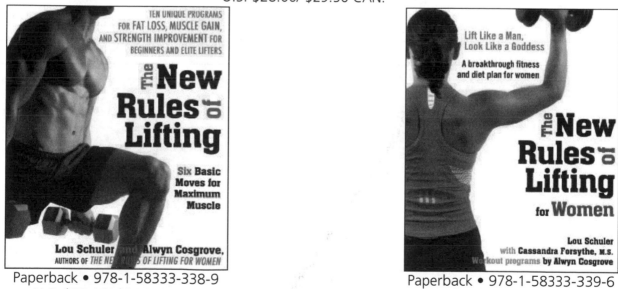